Vascular Access
for Bloodpurification Methods
and Catheter Technology

Edited by ROLF BAMBAUER

Rolf Bambauer (Ed.)

Vascular Access for Bloodpurification Methods and Catheter Technology

International Symposium
held at Homburg/Saar, FRG
November, 10-12, 1988

Sponsored by:
International Society for Artificial Organs (ISAO)
European Society for Artificial Organs (ESAO)

With 70 Figures and 72 Tables

Wolfgang Pabst Verlag

CIP Kurztitelaufnahme der Deutschen Bibliothek

Vascular access for bloodpurification methods and catheter technology : international symposium held at Homburg/Saar, FRG, November, 10-12, 1988 ; with 72 tables / Rolf Bambauer (ed.). Sponsored by: International Society for Artificial Organs (ISAO) ; European Society for Artificial Organs (ESAO). – Lengerich : Pabst 1992.
ISBN 3-928057-16-2
NE: Bambauer, Rolf [Hrsg.]

Printed in Germany

Publishing Management: Dr. Grund, Dr. Wender & Co., Saarbrücken, FRG
Printing and Binding: SDV Saarbrücker Druckerei und Verlag GmbH, Saarbrücken, FRG

ISBN 3-928057-16-2

Contents

Catheter Technology: Biocompatibility

Catheter Technology: Techniques

Peritoneal Access: Overview

Peritoneal Access: Clinical Applications

Therapeutic Plasma Exchange

Introduction

The International Symposium on "Vascular Access for Bloodpurification Methods and Catheter Technology", sponsored by the International Society of Artificial Organs (ISAO), European Society of Artificial Organs (ESAO) and the University of Saarland was held in Homburg/Saar, Federal Republic of Germany from 10th-12th November 1988. This International Symposium was part of an ongoing series of Symposia sponsored in the field of artificial organs especially in hemodialysis and apheresis techniques.

A very important part of these modern therapeutic methods is vascular access. Despite all technical innovations in infusion, transfusion therapies, hemodialysis and apheresis treatments the problem of finding a temporary or permanent vascular entry point appears to have no satisfactory solution. Temporary vascular access, in particular still presents considerable problems with handling, materials, intraluminal thrombosis, bacterial contamination, etc. In the past, there has been a tremendous effort by the industry, bioengineers, physicians etc. to develop new catheter systems like single lumen, double lumen large bore catheters, implantable catheters, catheters coated with heparin, biocarbon or other substances to minimize the side effects and complications and to achieve better biocompatibility. With new investigation methods like laboratory tests, scanning electron microscopy etc. the disadvantages and advantages of different catheters and their material can be better defined.

Since 1979 when I was first confronted with problems associated with vascular access in patients suffering from end stage renal failure, I introduced in our department the percutaneous puncturing of the internal jugular vein for placing a large bore catheter by applying the Seldinger technique. In the following years we made several improvements and developed with various companies new large bore catheters and contamination safeguards.

It is very difficult to realize new catheter concepts with the industry. As a physician I have been confronted with problems of the available catheters until today. Therefore we organized a special International Catheter Symposium, which was sponsored by the ISAO and the ESAO, to bring together all scientists working on this field, the industry, etc.

The aim of this International Symposium was to discuss the experiences of different vascular access methods, catheter technologies and new developments and strategies.

Approximately 100 attendees from FRG, other European countries, United States and Japan participated in the two day symposium. In eight different sessions about 40 papers were presented. The main topics were vascular access for blood-purification, catheter technology, biocompatibility, techniques, peritoneal access, clinical application and therapeutic plasma exchange. Most of the presentations summarized the experiences with double lumen or implantable catheters and new technologies. Others showed results of biocompatibility tests or scanning electron microscopy. In other sessions the results of new peritoneal access methods and clinical applications with small bore catheters were presented. In the last session some new results in therapeutic plasma exchange were offered.

All attendees were involved in critical discussions and a lot of statements were given. Most of the participants confirmed that the scientific level of this second International Symposium was very high and all scientists, physicians and bio-engineers were able to exchange ideas actively. The organization of this congress also provided us with useful experience.

I would like to thank Dr. Yukihiko Nosé who opened this International Symposium with his Festvortrag "Das Einfachste ist so wie das Vollkommene" and he closed the symposium with a summary of critical aspects and new impressions of catheter technology which indicate future trends.

Further I would like to thank warmly Dr. Paul S. Malchesky for his help in editing this Proceedings.

Last but not least I would like to thank Dr. Grund, Dr. Wender, Mr. Thieltges and the staff of the Arbeitsstelle für Literaturwissenschaftliche Datenverarbeitung of the Department of Germanic Studies, University of Saarland, Saarbrücken, for developing and adapting software in electronic data processing and publishing the scientific texts. This group is responsible for the layout and the technical aspects of publishing this Proceedings book.

Unfortunately the Proceedings are published late, but I hope not to late. It was very difficult to collect the manuscripts of all authors, some of them I am missing until today.

I hope that it will be possible in the future to use ISAO and ESAO symposia as a medium to contribute towards the development in various fields of artificial organs, as we have done for the second time here.

Homburg/Saar, November 10th, 1991 — Rolf Bambauer

List of Authors

AGISHI, T.
Department of Surgery, Kidney Center, Tokyo Women's Medical College, Tokyo, Japan

BAMBAUER, R.
Department of Nephrology, Med. Univ.-Klinik und Poliklinik, Universität des Saarlandes, Homburg/Saar, FRG

BASTERT, G.
Gynecological Department of the University Clinics Heidelberg, Heidelberg, FRG

DE BAZ, H.
see Panarello

BEELEN, R.
see Hombrouckx

BEHM, E.
see Schmitt

BEHREND, D.
Department of Internal Medicine, University of Rostock, FRG

BENEDIK, M.
see Ponikvar

BERKE, A.
Gambro GmbH, München, FRG

BOGAERT, A. M.
see Hombrouckx

BOHNDORF, K.
see Vorwerk

BOSCH, TH.
Nephrological Department, Medical Clinic I, Klinikum Großhadern, University of München, München, FRG

BRANDNER, P.
Gynecological Department, Med. Univ.-Klinik und Poliklinik, Universität des Saarlandes, Homburg/Saar, FRG

BREN, A.
Department of Nephrology, University Medical Center, Ljubljana, Yugoslavia

BROWN, G. S.
see Behrend

BUDDENHAGEN, F.
see Schmitt

CASCIANI, C.
see Morosetti

CHENG, C.-H.
see Lian

CHIARADIA, V.
see Panarello

DE CICCO, M.
see Panarello

ČIŽMAN , B.
see Ponikvar

DREWS, G.
see Behrend

DRINOVEC, J.
see Bren

FALKENHAGEN, D.
see Behrend

FRACASSO, A.
see Panarello

FUJITA, S.
see Agishi

DI GIOVANNA, F.
see Stalteri

DI GIULIO, S.
see Morosetti

GUBINA, M.
see Koselj

GUČEK, A.
Department of Nephrology, University Medical Center, Ljubljana, Yugoslavia

GÜNTHER, R. W.
see Vorwerk

D'HALLUIN, F.
see Hombrouckx

HAYASHI, T.
see Agishi

HEDBERG, B.
see Stegmayr

HELZEL, M. V.
Abteilung für Röntgen- und Strahlentherapie, Luitpold-Krankenhaus Würzburg, Würzburg, FRG

HITZSCHKE, B.
see Schmitt

HOENICH, N.
University of Newcastle, Medical School, Newcastle, UK

HOMBROUCKX, R.
Dialysis Unit, Kliniek Hogerlucht, Ronse, Belgium

HONDA, H.
see Agishi

HRUBÝ, M.
Department of Medicine, Charles University Medical School, Praha, CSFR

IVANOVICH, P.
V. A. Lakeside Hospital, North Western University, Chicago, USA

JUTZLER, G.
see Bambauer

KANDUS, A.
see Ponikvar

KAPLAN, S.
see Koselj

KAWAI, T.
see Agishi

KIMIKAWA, M.
see Agishi

KISTLER, D.
see Vorwerk

KITAJIMA, K.
see Agishi

KLINKMANN, H.
see Schmidt, R.

KOSELJ, M.
Department of Nephrology, University Medical Center, Ljubljana, Yugoslavia

KRACHT, M.
see Schmitt

KRAMANN, B.
Department of Radiodiagnostic, Med. Univ.-Klinik und Poliklinik, Universität des Saarlandes, Homburg/Saar, FRG

KRÖNUNG, G.
Chirurgische Universitätsklinik und Poliklinik Bonn, FRG

KUNDT, G.
see Schmitt

KURAJSKÝ, J.
see Hrubý

KVEDER, R.
see Varl

LAPČÍK, O.
see Hrubý

LARNO, L.
see Hombrouckx

LEROY, F.
see Hombrouckx

LIAN, J.-D.
Section of Nephrology, Department of Medicine, Taichung Veterans General Hospital, Taichung, Taiwan

LIČINA, A.
see Koselj

LINDIČ, J.
see Bren

LOIBL, U.
3rd Medical Department, Wilheminenspital, Vienna, Austria

LO PICCOLO, G.
see Stalteri

MALCHESKY, P. S.
see Naganuma

MALOVRH, M.
Department of Nephrology, University Medical Center, Ljubljana, Yugoslavia

MANGEL, E.
Department of Radiology and Renal Unit, Med. Klinik Innenstadt der Universität München, München, FRG

MANKER, W.
see Loibl

MANN, H.
see Vorwerk

DE MEESTER, J.
Department of Nephrology, University Hospital, Ghent, Belgium

MEISL, F.
see Loibl

MELONI, C.
see Morosetti

MESCHINI, L.
see Morosetti

MESTRES, P.
Department of Anatomy, Med. Univ.-Klinik und Poliklinik, Universität des Saarlandes, Homburg/Saar, FRG

MEYER-RIENECKER, H.
see Schmitt

MIYASHITA, C.
see Seyfert

MONTELEONE, F.
see Stalteri

MOROSETTI, M.
Clinica Chirurgica II, Universita di Roma, Roma, Italy

NAGANUMA, S.
Department of Artificial Organs, Cleveland Clinic Foundation, Cleveland (Ohio), USA

NEIS, K. J.
see Brandner

NOSÉ, Y.
Department of Artificial Organs, Cleveland Clinic Foundation, Cleveland (Ohio), USA

ONITSUKA, S.
see Agishi

OOBA, S.
see Agishi

OSANAI, K.
see Agishi

OSTEN, B.
see Schmidt, R.

OTA, K.
see Agishi

OZASA, S.
see Agishi

PALM, M.
see Schmitt

PANARELLO, G.
Department of Nephrology and Microbiology, Pordenone Hospital, Pordenone, Italy

PFEIFER, K. J.
see Mangel

PINDUR, G.
see Seyfert

PONIKVAR, R.
Department of Nephrology, University Medical Center, Ljubljana, Yugoslavia

PUTZKE, H.-P.
see Behrend

RINGOIR, S.
see Vanholder

SANDZEN, B.
see Stegmayr

SANTINI, G.
see Panarello

SAWADA, K.
see Naganuma

SCHERER, K.
see Kramann

SCHIFFL, H.
see Mangel

SCHMIDT, R.
Department of Internal Medicine, University of Rostock, FRG

SCHMIDT, W.
see Brandner

SCHMITT, E.
Department of Internal Medicine, University of Rostock, FRG

SEYFERT, U. T.
Department of Clinical Hemostaseology and Transfusion Medicine, Med. Univ.-Klinik und Poliklinik, Universität des Saarlandes, Homburg/Saar, FRG

SIEBERTH, H. G.
see Vorwerk

STALTERI, A.
Department of Nephrology, Sciacca Hospital, Sciacca, Italy

STEGMAYR, B.
Division of Nephrology, University Hospital, Umeå, Sweden

STEINBACH, K.
see Loibl

SUHADOLNIK-LIČINA, A.
see Ponikvar

SULKOVÁ, S.
see Hrubý

TACCONE-GALLUCCI, M.
see Morosetti

TERAOKA, S.
see Agishi

TESIO, F.
see Panarello

TESTA, V.
see Panarello

VÁLEK, A.
see Hrubý

VANHOLDER, R.
Department of Nephrology, University Hospital, Ghent, Belgium

VARL, J.
Department of Nephrology, University Medical Center, Ljubljana, Yugoslavia

VERREET, P. R.
Department of Surgery A, University of Düsseldorf, Düsseldorf, FRG

VORWERK, D.
Department of Diagnostic Radiology, Technical University of Aachen, Aachen, FRG

DE VOS, J. Y.
see Hombrouckx

WEBER, U.
Department of Nephrology, Med. Univ.-Klinik und Poliklinik, Universität des Saarlandes, Homburg/Saar, FRG

WENZEL, E.
see Seyfert

WIKDAHL, A. M.
see Stegmayr

WINKLER, R.
see Schmitt

Editorial

Y. Nosé

"Das Einfachste ist so wie das Vollkommene"

Recently, it is becoming more and more realistic to have a totally implantable cardiac prosthesis. Since this type of system is a quite complex artificial organ system involving a power system, an implantable feedback sensor, and a mechanical driving system, it is difficult to achieve the needed technologies together. Before we cover the technical problems to be overcome for successful totally implantable artificial organ systems, I would like to discuss five important fundamental philosophical points that need to be addressed to achieve this difficult goal.

The first is related to my experiences as a medical student in 1953. My Professor, Susumu Hozawa, Chairman, Department of Physiology, University of Hokkaido School of Medicine, told us many times in German "Das Einfachste ist so wie das Vollkommene", the simpler a physiological description is (of any given organ system), the closer it is to perfectly describing that system. Afterwards, I attended the University of Tokyo Postgraduate School of Engineering. At that time, Professor Shigeru Watanabe, Chairman of the Department of Mechanical Engineering, taught me the basic principles necessary for the simulation of human organs by engineering expressions. In principle, his philosophy seemed quite analogus to Professor Hozawa's since simpler equation systems are preferred over more complex arrays, and hence closer to perfection from his perspective. This same concept of "simplest is best" is even more relevant to medical doctors and engineers working together to generate new concepts in the field of totally implantable artificial organs.

The second point relevant to the successful development of organ replacement devices is the necessity for a clear definition of objectives. Sometimes even the definition of terms in these goals can be a point of confusion. One example is the definition of a permanently implantable artificial heart. For Dr. Kolff, any implant longer than six months is considered permanent. But for others longer than two years, or perhaps seven years, implantation is permanent.

Before we started our totally implantable ventricular assist program at the Cleveland Clinic ten years ago, we had clearly defined our definition of such a device. This was important, if the definition is different, the criteria and requirements are also different. By permanent, we mean fail-safe operation for two years, with 80 % reliability. The half-life of the system is 4.5 years. Failure in this case was defined as a pump flow less than two L/min for more than three min, traceable to pump performance.

In contrast, most of the already proven artificial organs such as pacemakers, heart valves, and so on are required to function effectively and safely for more than seven years. However, 25 years ago when the first implantable pacemaker was developed, the word permanent implied to anything longer than two years.

The key question remains, is there any permanent implantable artificial heart available now? If the definition is six months, certainly, yes. If the definition is two years, we believe it will be ready in a few years. If it is required for seven years, I dare say it is impossible to guarantee at this moment.

Even for a two-year system, the technical problems which must be overcome for a successful, totally implantable artificial organ system are numerous.

The system should be anatomically and biochemically compatible with surrounding tissues and blood. The implanted system should be durable and reliable during the expected operational period. Also, the implanted artificial organ should have effective and predictable performance.

The compatibility of the implant to the surrounding tissue and blood is, of course, extremely important. However, this is an extremely difficult task. Again and again we have been disappointed whenever we have gone against mother nature. This is because, basically, the human body was built to reject any kind of foreign invasion. Fighting against the recipient is not a good idea. So, if you cannot beat them, it is better to develop a method to join them. This is the third philosophical point I would like to stress.

For this reason, the "biolization" concept was introduced by our group in 1971 as a coating for blood-contacting surfaces of the implants. The coating of various surfaces by crosslinked gelatin, or other protein, renders it a seamless, hydrophilic, smooth biological surface. Such a surface has demonstrated excellent blood compatibility.

The fourth point I would like to stress is that the system we intend to develop should be as predictable as possible.

After implantation of the artificial heart, the recipient is believed to go through three stages. I believe this process would be similar with other surgical implants. Initially, the recipient does not know how to cope with the implant. (The first stage is the confusing stage.) The existing feedback systems of the body do not know how to function together with this device. Consequently, it is necessary for the remaining physiological feedback systems to adapt, somehow, to whatever mechanism was implanted. However, after some time, we believe the recipient will learn to cope with the implant. The mode of control, though, is quite different from the existing feedback systems with the original natural organ. In general, the recipient and the implant are fighting together to establish their coexistence. (The second stage is the fighting stage.) Usually the confusion stage is for two to three hours and the fighting stage will last for two to four weeks. If the implant system is simple and its performance is quite predictable, the fighting stage becomes shorter and this phase is not as serious. However, if the implanted system is not performing in a predictable fashion, death of the recipient usually results. If the patient survives the fighting stage, he will, one hopes, make a smooth transition to the "live together" stage (the third stage). In the case of cardiac prostheses, during this fighting stage typically abnormal physiologies are revealed. These include an increase in peripheral resistance, an increase in circulatory blood volume, and an increase in the venous pressure together with increased levels of catecholamine. However, these are transient phenomena and will be over usually within three weeks after implantation. So again, any of the surgically implantable systems must be as simple and predictable as possible for the recipient.

Currently the most feasible implantable artificial organ systems are those that are electrically powered. Power supply and power transmission technologies are well established. Intrinsic sensors which function fail-safe for over two years are available. Also a reliable transcutaneous diagnostic signal transmission is feasible. At this time, we believe the truly feasible, permanently implantable system should be either electro-mechanical or electro-hydraulic.

Unfortunately, when it is an electro-chemical system that is required for the metabolic artificial organs (those which regulate input and output of metabolites), the conventional methods, developed for extracorporeal systems, are not feasible. It is therefore necessary to develop unconventional methods which are different in concept from those currently in existence. This is the fifth point I would like to stress.

One good example is the development of an implantable artificial kidney. The hemodialyzer was designed to function most effectively in an extracorporeal environment, not in the body. In other words, completely different concepts are necessary to make the totally implantable metabolic system a reality.

Vascular Access for Bloodpurification: Acute Vascular Access

Risk Factors for Blood Access Trouble in Maintenance Hemodialysis

T. Agishi, K. Osanai, T. Kawai, S. Ozasa, T. Hayashi, M. Kimikawa,
S. Fujita, S. Onitsuka, K. Kitajima, K. Ota

Abstract

Current status and past history of the blood access for maintenance hemodialysis were investigated in the patients who have been chronically dialyzed in our dialysis facility and the affiliated institutions in an attempt to clarify the possible risk factors for the problems and the complications. A total of the 707 patients were entered into the study. The multifactorial analysis was made between individual parameters for the possible risk factors such as age, sex, hemodialysis term, original disease and blood pressure and for the present blood access status such as type, site, the number of the operations, difficulty in needle puncture, blood flow during dialysis and the complications. The analytical results indicated older age, female, longer hemodialysis term, diabetes and collagen disease as original diseases and low blood pressure are the risk factors for the blood access troubles with statistical significance.

Introduction

Presence of the blood access offering reliable and sufficient blood flow is a fundamental requisite for the well-being of the chronic hemodialysis patients. However, its condition is not always easily maintained to be satisfactory. Therefore, analysis of the possible risk factors which may threaten the status of the blood access is considered to be worthwhile because it may present a clue to prevent the malfunctioning or the complications of the blood access.

Materials and Methods

Current status and past history of the blood access of the patients who have been dialyzed in the dialysis unit of Kidney Center, Tokyo Women's Medical College and in the affiliated institutions were investigated. For this purpose, a questionnaire including both a list of the background factors postulated as the possible risk factors and a list of the present condition and a past history of the blood access(es)

Table 1. Possible Risk Factors.

age (years old)	original diseases
0 - 9	chronic glomerulonephritis
10 - 19	chronic pyelonephritis
20 - 39	diabetes mellitus
40 - 59	polycystic kidney
60 - 79	collagen disease
80 -	unclear
sex	others (VUR, hydronephrosis, nephrosis, gout, pregnant kidney,
male	Barter's syndrome, hypoplasia purpura)
female	
HD duration (D, years)	blood pressure (mm Hg)
$D \leq 1$	< 99
$1 < D \leq 3$	100 - 149
$3 < D \leq 6$	150 - 199
$6 < D \leq 12$	$200 <$
$12 < D \leq 15$	
$15 < D$	

postulated as the blood access status was sent to each institution and filled in by the dialysis doctors or nurses. Lists of those factors with more detailed items are presented in Table 1 and 2.

An analysis was made trying to find out a statistically significant correlation between each of the itemized risk factors and each of the blood access status parameters.

Statistical significance was evaluated by a student t-test between the individualized items.

Results

A total of 707 patient data was collected. Statistical significance was classified as * for $0.02 < p \leq 0.05$, ** for $0.01 < p \leq 0.02$ and *** for $p \leq 0.01$.

1. Factors influencing the type of the blood access are indicated in Table 3.
2. Factors influencing the site of the blood access are indicated in Table 4.
3. Factors influencing the number of the blood access operations are indicated in Table 5.
4. Factors influencing the difficulty in puncturing the blood access are indicated in Table 6.
5. Factors influencing blood flow during hemodialysis are indicated in Table 7.
6. Factors influencing complications of the blood access are indicated in Table 8.

Table 2. Blood Access Status.

type of present blood access	duration of present blood access
internal shunt	– 6 months
external shunt	– 1 year
graft	– 3 years
arterial superficialization	– 5 years
	more than 5 years
site of present blood access	type of longest blood access survival
forearm (primary)	internal shunt
forearm (others)	external shunt
elbow-upper arm	graft
thigh	arterial superficialization
others	others
number of operations (times)	
1	
2	
3	
4	
$5 \leq$ No. < 10	
$10 \leq$ No.	
longest duration of blood access	complications of blood access
	internal shunt
– 6 months	infection
– 1 year	thrombus formation
– 3 years	sore thumb
– 5 years	steal syndrome
more than 5 years	aneurysm
	others
difficulty in puncturing	graft
easy	infection
moderate	thrombus formation
difficult	steal syndrome
	lymph edema
	others
blood flow (ml/min)	
- 99	
100 - 149	
150 - 199	
200 -	

Discussion

Correlation between the possible risk factors and the status of the blood access was statistically investigated in the questionnaire data of the patients who have been chronically hemodialyzed in our affiliated institutions. Since the blood accesses of almost all of these patients have been controlled under an identical treatment concept, the analysis results are expected to offer a common medical meaning.

Table 3. Type of Blood Access.

– Arterial superficialization is more frequent in > 60 year old patients ***.
– Graft or arterial superficialization is more frequent in female patients ***. Internal shunt is in male patients ***.
– Graft is more frequent in patients > 15 years HD **.

*: $0.02 < p \leq 0.05$, **: $0.01 < p \leq 0.02$, ***: $p \leq 0.01$

Table 4. Site of Blood Access.

– In > 60 year old patients, primary internal shunt is less frequent *. In > 80 year old patients, blood access is created more frequently in elbow-upper arm **.
– In females, blood access other than primary internal shunt is more frequent ***.
– In patients hemodialyzed for 1 - 6 years, primary internal shunt is more popular **.
– In collagen disease patients, primary internal shunt is less frequent ***.

*: $0.02 < p \leq 0.05$, **: $0.01 < p \leq 0.02$, ***: $p \leq 0.01$

Table 5. Number of Blood Access Operations.

– In patients of age 60 - 79 years old, more than 4 operations have been more frequently done ***.
– Patients operated only once are more in male *** and for < 1 year HD duration ***.
– Patients operated more than 11 times are significantly more among patients for > 9 year HD duration **.
– Patients operated more than 4 times are more among diabetes ***.
– Patients with 100 - 199 mmHg blood pressure have undergone only one operation **.
– Diabetes and collagen disease patients have undergone more operations than chronic glomerulonephritis patients ***.
– Patients with < 99 mmHg blood pressure have undergone 4 operations **.

*: $0.02 < p \leq 0.05$, **: $0.01 < p \leq 0.02$, ***: $p \leq 0.01$

The analysis results can be interpreted as follows:

The type of the blood access: Arterial superficialization is chosen in the older patients in order to avoid an overload to the heart. The degree of the injury of the blood access proceeds faster in the female than the male. A graft implantation is the second choice after an internal shunt has been seriously destroyed by the numerous repetitions of the punctures.

The site of the blood access: The blood access locates more in the elbow and the upper arm in the aged patients probably due to the difficulty in creation or complications of the blood access in the forearm. The male and the shorter-term patients are dialyzed using a primary internal shunt. In the patients with the collagen disease, a primary internal shunt is hard to be created or maintained due to an angitic lesion or complications which will be discussed later in the item of the complications.

Table 6. Difficulty in Puncturing Blood Access.

- "Easy" patients are more in the 40 - 59 year of age group ***.
- "Moderate" or "difficult" patients are more in female ***.
- In diabetes patients, "easy" or "moderate" are less compared to chronic glomerulonephritis patients ***.
- "Easy" patients are more in 100 - 199 mmHg blood pressure patients **.

*: $0.02 < p \leq 0.05$, **: $0.01 < p \leq 0.02$, ***: $p \leq 0.01$

The number of the blood access operations: The number of the blood access operations increases in the aged and the longer-term hemodialysis patients Diabetes and collagen disease as the original disease and low blood pressure are the risk factors for the blood access troubles.

Difficulty in puncturing the blood access: The male, the middle aged and the moderate blood pressure patients have the easily puncturable blood accesses, while the diabetes patients have difficulty in puncturing.

Blood flow during hemodialysis: The younger patients dialyzed for intermediate-term with moderate blood pressure and introduced to dialysis with chronic glomerulonephritis have well-functioning blood accesses.

Table 7. Blood Flow during Hemodialysis.

- In patients of age 20 - 39 years old, > 200 ml/min is more easily obtained ***.
- In patients dialyzed for 9 - 15 years, > 200 ml/min is more easily obtained ***.
- In chronic glomerulonephritis patients, > 200 ml/min is more easily obtained ***.
- In patients with 100 - 199 mmHg blood pressure, > 200 ml/min is more easily obtained ***.

*: $0.02 < p \leq 0.05$, **: $0.01 < p \leq 0.02$, ***: $p \leq 0.01$

Complications in the blood access: In regard to internal shunts, diabetes and polycystic kidney disease as an original disease are more risky for thrombus formation compared to chronic glomerulonephritis. Steal syndrome tends to develop longer-term hemodialysis patients. Aneurysm more likely occurs in collagen disease patients probably due to vascular fragility by angitis and the previous steroid administration.

Conclusions

Most of the risk factors herein pointed out are supposed to be risky in routine practice. However, there have been no data available which have been statistically analyzed.

Table 8. Complications in Blood Access.

Internal shunt:
– Incidence of thrombus formation is diabetes, polycystic kidneys > collagen disease > chronic glomerulonephritis *.
– Steal syndrome more frequently occurs in patients dialyzed for 12 - 15 years **.
– Aneurysm more frequently occurs in collagen disease patients than in diabetes or polycystic kidney patients *.
Graft:
– Thrombus formation occurs less frequently in chronic pyelonephritis or collagen disease patients than in chronic glomerulonephritis patients *.

*: $0.02 < p \leq 0.05$, **: $0.01 < p \leq 0.02$, ***: $p \leq 0.01$

In conclusion, older age, female, longer hemodialysis term, diabetes and collagen disease as an original disease and low blood pressure are the risk factors for the blood access trouble in chronic dialysis patients.

Complications in Vascular Access Device Treatment

T. AGISHI, T. HAYASHI, H. HONDA, S. OOBA, S. TERAOKA, K. OTA

Abstract

Intraarterial infusion of the anticancer drugs (IIAD) is a choice of treatment to be taken into consideration for the inoperable cancers. Usage of a vascular access device (VAD) which is subcutaneously implanted and delivers the percutaneously injected drugs to the cancer bearing organ via the feeding artery has been becoming popular in the IIAD. As clinical usefulness of this system is such as reported elsewhere, complications in the VAD treatment are herein reported. A total of 85 VADs has been implanted in 79 patients in our department and in the affiliated institutions. A whole VAD system was implanted through a laparotomy in 35 cases whereas a catheter of the VAD was inserted into the targeted artery via the femoral artery by a modified Seldinger's technique and connected with a reservoir in 50 cases. Complications encountered were as follows: occlusion of the system in 15 cases (17.6 %), local hematoma in seven cases (8.2 %), wound dehiscence in three cases (3.5 %), drug leakage in six cases (7.1 %), infection of the wound in four cases (4.7 %) and ulcer formation in four cases (4.7 %). However, most of the complications are supposed to be avoided by being acquainted with the skills to manipulate the VAD system.

Introduction

Intraarterial infusion of the anticancer drugs (IIAD) is the treatment of choice to be taken into consideration for inoperable cancers. Recently, a vascular access device (VAD) which is subcutaneously implanted and delivers the percutaneously injected drugs to the cancer bearing organ via the feeding artery has been devised and becoming popularly used in IIAD for the purpose of targeting therapy. As clinical usefulness of this system is such as reported elsewhere, complications in the VAD treatment are to be herein discussed.

Materials and Methods

A vascular access device (VAD) is an implantable system composed of a fine silicone rubber catheter (OD 2.0 mm, ID 1.0 mm) and a volcano-shaped reservoir. They communicate each other with a common internal lumen. Therefore, drugs

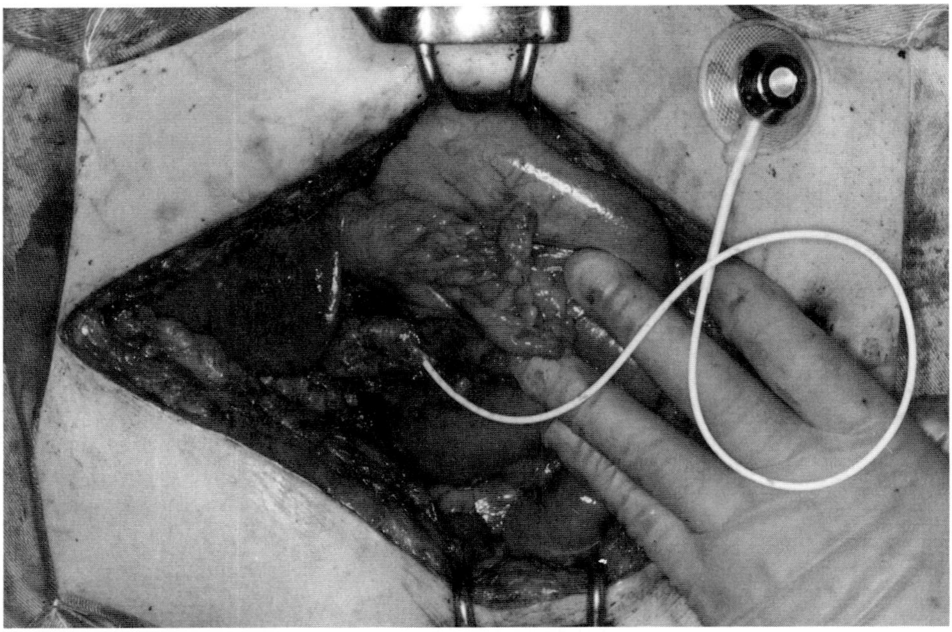

Fig. 1. Vascular access device.

percutaneously injected into a lumen of the subcutaneously positioned reservoir through a silicone rubber central plug are delivered to the cancer bearing organ via a catheter indwelling in the feeding artery (Fig. 1).

For insertion of the catheter, an operative or a modified Seldinger's catheter technique is currently applicable.

An operative insertion is indicated for secure positioning of a catheter tip while a modified Seldinger's one is done in patients in whom the feeding artery can not be operatively reached mainly because of the tumor invasion or the severe general condition. However, the latter has been becoming popular for technical easiness.

A venedotomy technique is utilized to the operatively exposed artery for an operative insertion of the catheter in continuity with the subcutaneously implanted reservoir.

On the other hand, a catheter inserted either by a venedotomy technique or a direct puncture to the femoral artery is advanced up to the targeted artery in a similar manner to the angiographic technique for the modified Seldinger's technique. The infusion catheter was afterwards connected with the separately implanted reservoir.

In our institution, most of the patients who have undergone this targeted cancer therapy have been treated in combination with local hyperthermia. Although clinical usefulness of this combined modality of the therapy has been confirmed and reported elsewhere [1, 2], the main subject of this article is not directed to discuss the clinical efficacy, but reliability and the problems of this implantable catheter treatment.

A total of 85 VADs has been implanted in 79 patients for the purpose of chemotherapy in a variety of extensive cancers since April, 1984 in our department and the affiliated institutions (Table 1). Sixty-one patients had liver tumors either with primary hepatocellular carcinomas or metastatic hepatic carcinomas.

Table 1. Original diseases for VAD implantations.

Vascular Access Device Implantations	
Original Diseases	Number of Patients
liver tumor	61
primary hepatocellular cancer	24
metastatic hepatic cancer	37
pelvic tumor	14
prostate cancer	8
uroepitheliar cancer	6
others	4
total	79

85 implantations in 79 patients
male: 61, female: 18, 17-85 years old

The VADs were implanted operatively in 35 patients and by the modified Seldinger's technique in 50 patients.

38 VADs were implanted for an earlier period from April, 1984 to December, 1986 and 47 for a later period from January, 1987 to October, 1988.

Injection of the anticancer agents was initiated after the wound healing was completed and performed either in a one-shot manner or twice a week or in a continuous manner using a small portable infusion pump.

Results

Patency of the system

32 months of survival was achieved in one patient by this treatment. The longest patient period of the system was 24 months. When a patient died, a VAD was calculated as being occluded.

An average patent rate of the system, which means that the system was usable for chemotherapy, was 54.3 % (19 patent out of 35 VADs) in the operative catheter insertions compared to 40.0 % (20 patent out of 50 VADs) in the modified Seldinger's insertions 12 months after the implantations. The difference between the two became smaller thereafter (Fig. 2).

An average patency of 28.9 % was maintained of the system (11 patent out of 38 VADs) for the earlier period from April, 1984 to December, 1986 compared

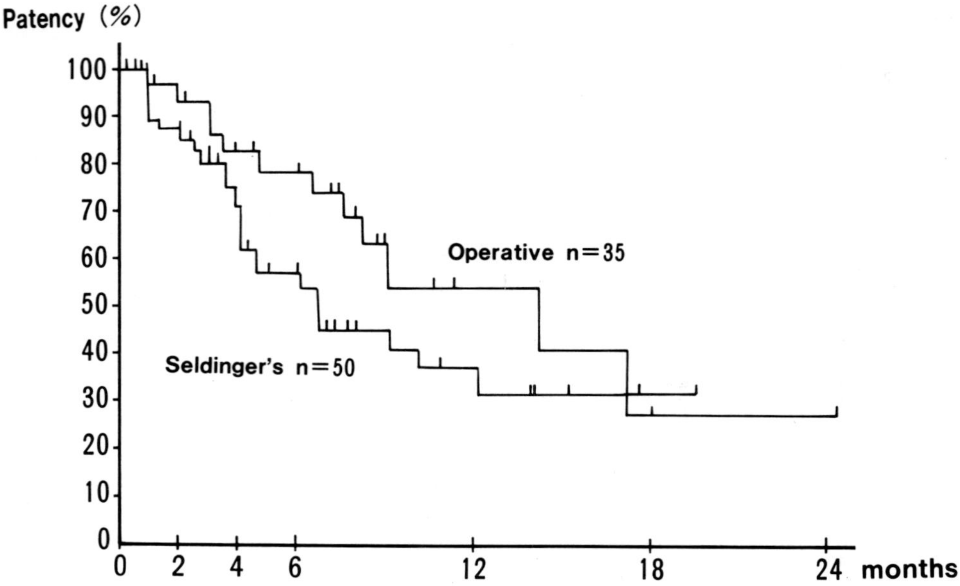

Fig. 2. VAD patency (implementation technique).

to 63.8 % (30 patent out of 47 VADs) for the later period from January, 1987 to October, 1988 12 months after the implantations. The difference in the patency remained thereafter (Fig. 3).

Complications in VAD implantations

1. Occlusion of VAD. Occlusion means that the system occludes and the injection has to be interrupted even though still desired. It occurred in 15 instances out of the 85 implantations (17.6 %).
2. Local troubles at the site of the VAD implantations such as hematoma, wound dehiscence, drug leakage from the reservoir and infection were observed.

Table 2. Complications in VAD implantations.

Complications	Cases	%
occlusion of VAD	15	17.6
local trouble		
hematoma	7	8.2
wound dehiscene	3	3.5
drug leakage	6	7.1
infection	4	4.7
others		
ulcer	4	4.7
disconnection of VAD	1	1.2
vascular occlusion	3	3.5
plug leakage	1	1.2

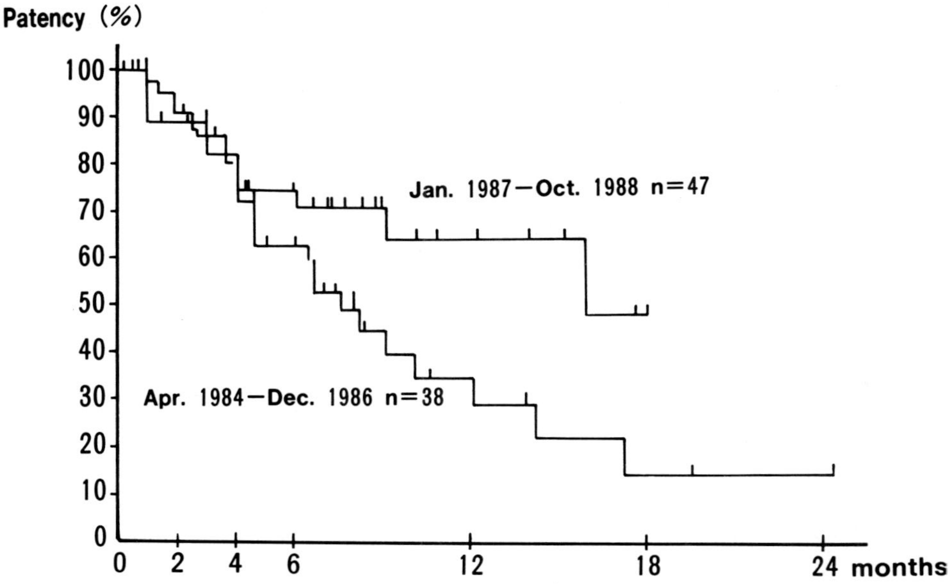

Fig. 3. VAD patency (period of study).

3. Ulcer formation was found in four cases. Two were in the duodenum in a treatment course of the liver tumor probably due to insufficient blood supply from the gastroduodenal artery while two were in the perineal region in a treatment of the prostate. Disconnection of the system occurred at an early stage due to a mistaken percutaneous puncture of catheter with a needle Vascular occlusion occurred in three cases. Plug leakage occurred in one case (Table 2).

Discussion

Recently a novel trend has been becoming prominent in therapeutic technology. It is so-called "target therapy" in which a treatment is aimed to be focused particularly on the diseased tissue or organ in order to increase the cost-effectiveness performance and to avoid the unnecessary side-effects.

Intraarterial infusion of the anticancer agents is a method corresponding to this concept. Until recently, it had been only performed via a percutaneously indwelling catheter. Although a newly devised VAD system has been shown advantageous over a percutaneously indwelling catheter and clinical effectiveness of the cancer treatment with this system has been already reported, reliability and the clinical problems in usage of the system have not been described.

Eleven Years Experience with Continuous Central Venous Catheter Hemodialysis: a Review

R. VANHOLDER, N. HOENICH, S. RINGOIR

Abstract

The morbidity and mortality of hemodialysis by continuous internal central venous catheterization in the subclavian, internal jugular and femoral positions are reviewed. A follow-up study was performed over 11 years (1405 catheterizations). The most frequent complications were inadequate flow (10.7 %), bacteremia (5.3 %) and inadvertent withdrawal (4.2 %). The overall complication rate was 25.3 %. Traumatic complications such as pneumothorax, hemothorax, air embolism or retroperitoneal bleeding were extremely rare (23 in total – 1.6 %). Three subgroups were related to 702 subclavian, 236 internal jugular and 467 femoral catheterizations. The overall complication rate was similar for each of the above mentioned insertion sites. Inadvertent withdrawal was the only complication observed more frequently in the internal jugular than in the subclavian or the femoral position (10.8 vs 4.3 and 2.5 %; $p < 0.01$). Flow problems were significantly more frequent in patients with femoral catheterization (16.4 %), compared to the internal jugular (7.0 %) and the subclavian position (7.8 %). No fatal complications were observed after subclavian and deep jugular catheterization. One fatality after femoral catheterization was due to a deconnection, followed by shock and death. These data suggest that, if applied correctly, the morbidity and mortality of central venous catheter dialysis can be kept extremely low. The most disturbing complications (inadequate flow, bacteremia) can be related to the bioincompatibility of the catheter polymers.

Introduction

Central venous catheterization allows immediate and easy access to the vascular bed for hemodialysis.

In our unit, central venous catheters have been used as a vascular access since 1977. Catheters have been used in the subclavian, internal jugular and femoral position, as previously described [1-3].

This paper mainly evaluates the general characteristics and the complication profile for these different insertion sites.

Patients and Methods

A follow-up study was conducted at the University Hospital of Ghent. Catheters were only inserted by staff physicians. Up to 1981, nonradiopaque dialysis catheters (Femoral catheter, Extracorporeal Medical Specialties, King of Prussia, Pa., USA) were introduced according to the Seldinger technique, after prior insertion of a radiopaque polyethylene catheter, at least in the subclavian and the internal jugular positions. During the last seven years, radiopaque polyurethane catheters (Vas-Cath, Gambro, Lund, Sweden) were used. Subclavian catheters were introduced via the infraclavicular Aubaniac [4] pathway, as described earlier [3]. Jugular catheterization has been performed only during the last five years of the study. Femoral catheters were inserted according to general conditions, but were kept in place continuously. Thus, they were not repositioned at each dialysis, as is done usually.

Hemodialysis was performed using a single-needle procedure (BL760, Bellco, Mirandola, Italy). To maintain patency of the catheter, continuous infusion systems were connected to it, or when this was not necessary, the catheter was flushed with saline and filled with heparin.

The catheters were maintained in place until further treatment became unnecessary (at recovery of normal physiological functions, after the puncture of an adequate fistula or after initiation of peritoneal dialysis) unless death occurred or unless the catheter was withdrawn because of problems.

Complications were registered and could be subdivided in traumatic problems, immediately after insertion (puncture of the subclavian, carotid or femoral artery, hemothorax, hemoperitoneum, pneumothorax, etc.) and of problems occurring later in the treatment course (inadequate flow, catheter-related bacteremia, tear of the catheter wall, disconnection, deep venous thrombosis).

Inadequate flow was defined as the impossibility to build up a sufficient blood flow in the dialysis system, necessitating replacement of the catheter.

Catheter bacteremia was diagnosed if an overtly febrile state was found in the absence of any other frank reason for infection, and/or if a semiquantitative culture of the catheter tip yielded more than 15 colonies per tip, and the same species was recovered from blood cultures.

Clinical internal venous thrombosis was diagnosed in the presence of limb edema on the catheterization side, together with phlebographic evidence of venous thrombosis.

Results

The frequency at which central vein catheter dialysis was used in our unit is illustrated in Table 1. These catheters were used in a total number of 9,913 dialyses or related procedures. In total 1405 catheters were inserted in 1013 patient procedures. These catheters were subdivided between 3 different insertion sites: subclavian (n = 702), internal jugular (n = 236) and femoral (n = 467). They were inserted in acute conditions in 686 cases and in chronic conditions in 719 cases.

Table 1. Central Vein Catheter Hemodialysis.

Total number of		Insertion sites		Conditions	
Dialyses	9,913	Subclavian	702	Acute	686
Catheters	1,405	Int. Jugular	236	Chronic	719
Pat. Episodes	1,013	Femoral	467		

Overall follow-up lasted 21 029 days (15.0 d/cath.). Follow-up under acute conditions was much shorter than under chronic conditions (4.9 and 24.5 d/cath respectively).

The different complications that were registered in a prospective way are illustrated in Table 2. Some complications, such as inadequate flow and bacteremia, may be defined as biocompatibility related. Others, such as hemothorax, hemopericardium etc. are typically traumatic.

Table 2. Complications Registered.

Inadequate flow°	Arterial puncture*
Bacteremia°	Hemothorax*
Inadvertent withdrawal	Deep venous thrombosis
Bleeding	Pneumothorax*
Tear catheter wall	Local pain
Disconnection	Air embolism*
Local Hematoma*	Pulmonary embolism

° : biocompatibility
* : traumatic

The general distribution of the major complications is illustrated in Table 3. In general most complications look rather trivial. Most frequent problems are those of inadequate flow and bacteremia, together responsible for 16.0 % of the registered complications. Inadvertent withdrawal occurs in 4.2 % of the cases. Traumatic complications are relatively rare, and are observed only at a frequency of 1.6 %. Comparing the different insertion sites, the overall complication incidence is similar and in the range of 25 % for the subclavian, internal jugular or femoral positions. However, if complications are considered separately, traumatic problems occur significantly less frequently in the femoral (0.5 %) vs the subclavian position (2.35 % – $p < 0.025$).

As far as non traumatic complications are concerned, no significant differences are observed, except for a somewhat higher incidence of inadvertent withdrawal in the deep jugular position (10.8 % vs 4.3 and 2.5 % for subclavian and femoral position – $p < 0.01$).

Also, flow problems were more frequent in patients with femoral catheterization (16.4 %) compared to the internal jugular (7.0 %) and the subclavian position (7.8 %).

Subclavian vein or superior vena cava occlusion was only registered if it was clinically positive, i.e. in the presence of ipsilateral limb edema and radiologically proven venous thrombosis. In total, this complication was only registered in 4 cases, all of them after a prolonged use of central vein catheters (> 3 months) in teflon.

No fatal complications were observed after subclavian and internal jugular catheterization. One fatality after femoral catheterization was due to a deconnection, followed by shock and death.

Table 3. Overall Complications.

	Number	%
Inadequate flow	151	10.7
Bacteremia	75	5.3
Inadvertent withdrawal	59	4.2
Traumatic	23	1.6
Other complications	47	3.3
Total	355	25.3

Discussion

The present paper reviews the overall experience in our unit with central vein catheters for hemodialysis. In total, more than 1400 catheters were inserted, corresponding to more than 1000 patient episodes. This approach allowed immediate treatment when necessary.

The present study evaluates the overall frequency of complications. An incidence of ±25 % may seem high, but it must be stressed that rather trivial problems like inadequate flow and inadvertent withdrawal were equally taken into consideration and composed the majority of the encountered complications. Although less important, inadequate flow may influence dialysis adequacy; it is obviously a bioincompatibility problem, related to catheter thrombogenicity. Another frequent complication, bacteremia, is also bioincompatibility related; more specifically, it may depend on the affinity of catheter material towards bacteria. Bacteremia may in rare cases give rise to a fatal outcome [1].

In general, complication profiles of different insertion sites are not dramatically divergent. Traumatic complications occur somewhat less frequent in the femoral position. It should be stressed, however, that we use these femoral catheters in a continuous way, and that they are not withdrawn and reinserted at each dialysis, as is done currently. This might have decreased the incidence of traumatic complications.

A somewhat disturbing complication is deep venous thrombosis, that was first described by our own group [3], and that seems especially related to a prolonged use of teflon catheters. It is important to stress that the clinical penetrance of this complication is extremely low, at least in our hands. Nevertheless incidence of this problem should be kept to a minimum, by using biocompatible material and by maintaining catheters in place for as short periods as possible. If a prolonged treatment is expected, alternative solutions, like Hickman catheters should be preferred.

In conclusion, our data indicate that central vein catheterization remains a valuable access method, especially in urgent situations. The complication profile shows no major differences between insertion sites. The most frequent complications are rather trivial, and seem to be related to the bioincompatibility of catheter materials, an aspect that often has been neglected.

Deep venous thrombosis with clinical penetrance is more exceptional as is generally believed, but should be avoided by limiting the duration of continuous catheter insertion. If longer treatment periods are expected, alternative methods like Hickman catheters should be preferred.

References

[1] VANHOLDER, R., N. A. HOENICH, S. RINGOIR: Morbidity and mortality of central venous catheter hemodialysis: a review of 10 years' experience. *Nephron* 47: 274-279 (1987).

[2] VANHOLDER, R. C., S. RINGOIR: Percutaneous femoral vessel cannulation for hemodialysis pp. 129-152. In: ANDREUCCI, V. E. (ed.): Vascular and peritoneal access for dialysis. Kleuver Academic Publ., Boston 1989.

[3] VANHOLDER, R., N. LAMEIRE, J. VERBANCK, R. VAN RATTINGHE, M. KUNNEN, S. RINGOIR: Complications of subclavian catheter hemodialysis: A 5-year prospective study in 257 consecutive patients. *Int. J. Artif. Organs* 5: 297-303 (1982).

[4] AUBANIAC, R.: L'injection intraveineuse sousclaviculaire: avantages et technique. *Presse méd* 60: 1456 (1952).

Eight Years Experience with Hemodialysis Catheters for Plasma Exchange Therapy

A. GUČEK, J. DRINOVEC, R. PONIKVAR, J. VARL, M. MALOVRH, A. BREN

Abstract

From March 1980 to June 1988 1472 plasma exchange therapies (PE) have been performed in our Center. Different vascular access techniques were used. 1076 hemodialysis (HD) femoral catheters were used for one procedure only and four catheters were maintained in place for 4-11 days (mean 7.8 ± 3.3). 12 subclavian catheters were inserted six without and six with subcutaneous tunnel and remained inserted two to 44 days (mean 16 ± 14). Side effects were rare with femoral catheters, only in 2.47 % (27 complications/1080 femoral catheters). Arterial punctures were observed in 1 % (11/1080), local hematomas in 0.27 % (3/1080), retroperitoneal hematoma 0.09 % (1/1080), local infections in 0.27 % (3/1080). Subclavian catheters had a higher complication rate, 41.5 % (five complications/12 subclavian catheters). There were unsuccessful cannulation in 8.3 % (1/12), local infections in 16.6 % (2/12) and sepsis in 16.6 % (2/12). There were no fatal complications, hemothorax or pneumothorax. The most serious complications were septicemia, exclusively with subclavian catheters inserted without subcutaneous tunnel.

Introduction

There is information concerning the frequency of complications of vascular access for hemodialysis (HD) [1-3] but the information is limited for plasma exchange therapy (PE). When peripheral vein cannulation is problematical the large vein percutaneous cannulation allows immediate access to the vascular bed for PE. This paper evaluates the frequency of complications of different HD catheters for PE in our unit.

Patients and Methods

A follow-up study from March 1980 to June 1988 was performed. 1472 PE have been performed in 108 patients, 55 females and 53 males, aged two months to

Table 1. Complication rate HD catheters for plasma exchange therapy.

Complication	HD catheter			
	Femoral cath. (No. 1080)		Subclavian cath. (No. 12)	
	No.	%	No.	%
Arterial puncture	11	1	0	0
Unsuccessful cannulation	8	0.75	1	8.3
Local hematoma	3	0.27	0	0
Retroperitoneal hematoma	1	0.09	0	0
Hemothorax	0	0	0	0
Pneumothorax	0	0	0	0
Thrombosis	1	0.09	0	0
Local infection	3	0.27	2	16.6
Sepsis	0	0	2	16.6
Fatal	0	0	0	0
Total	27	2.47	5	41.5

72 years (mean 33 ± 19.4). Different vascular access techniques were used: HD femoral catheter and peripheral vein in 1015 PE (69.0 %), HD subclavian catheter and peripheral vein in 78 PE (5.3 %), two peripheral veins in 242 PE (16.4 %), HD femoral catheter (single needle) in 85 PE (5.8 %), HD subclavian catheter (single needle) in 20 PE (1.4 %), A-V fistula in 27 PE (1.8 %) and A-V shunt in five PE (0.3 %). Catheters were inserted by Seldinger technique into the femoral or subclavian vein. We used wide-bore single lumen catheters: femoral (Extracorporeal teflon 360 × 2.0 mm, Deseret teflon 133 × 2.1 mm) and subclavian (Vas-Cath teflon 150 × 1.8 mm, Vas-Cath teflon 200 × 1.8 mm, Vas-Cath polyurethane 200 × 1.8 mm). 1076 femoral catheters were used for one procedure only and four catheters were maintained in place for 4-11 days (mean 7.8 ± 3.3). 12 subclavian catheters were inserted via the infraclavicular way, six without and six with subcutaneous tunnel. Chest radiographs were obtained in all patients to control position of catheters. Subclavian catheters remained inserted permanently two to 44 days (mean 16 ± 14).

Table 2. HD catheters for plasma exchange therapy.

Type of catheter	Number of plasma exchanges	Number of catheters	Complications of catheters	
			No	%
Femoral	1100	1080	27	2.47
Subclavian	98	12	5	41.5
nontunneled	78	6	3	24.9
tunneled	20	6	1	8.3

Results

The complication profiles are listed in Table 1 and Table 2. No fatal complications were registered. Sepsis was observed in nontunneled subclavian catheters ($2/6 = 33.3\,\%$). HD femoral catheters were associated with a low incidence of complications.

Conclusions

- Plasma exchanges were not limited by vascular access.
- When peripheral vein cannulation was problematical the large vein percutaneous cannulation allowed immediate access to the vascular bed. Side effects were rare and were not life threatening.
- HD femoral catheters were associated with a low incidence of complications.
- The most serious complications were sepsis exclusively with subclavian catheters inserted without subcutaneous tunnel.
- We suggest that HD femoral catheters should either be removed after each procedure or subclavian catheters placed through subcutaneous tunnel for permanent use.

References

[1] Erben, J., J. Kvasnicka, J. Bastecky, et al.: Long-term experience with the technique of subclavian and femoral vein cannulation in hemodialysis. *Artif. Organs* 3: 241-244 (1979).

[2] Uldall, P. R.: Subclavian cannulation for hemodialysis: the present state of the art. *Artif. Organs* 6: 73-76 (1982).

[3] Vanholder, R., N. A. Hoenich, S. Ringoir: Morbidity and mortality of central venous catheter hemodialysis: a review of 10 years experience. *Nephron* 47: 274-279 (1987).

Complications of Vascular Access in Chronic Hemodialysis: A Retrospective Study

U. LOIBL, W. MANKER, F. MEISL, K. STEINBACH

Abstract

In patients on chronic hemodialysis, complications of vascular access remain one of the most substantial problems. Therefore fistula complications of 94 patients (41 female, 53 male; mean age 61 years, range 19-83 years) with a mean duration of hemodialysis of 40 months per patient (range 3-200 months) were evaluated retrospectively.

121 fistulae with a primary function of > 3 months (78 Cimino, 23 Goretex, 10 saphena, five basilaris, and five homologous venous transplants) were evaluated: mean duration of function 43 ± 11 months, mean interval up to the first complication 33 ± 14 months.

Table 1.

Complications		Revision	Loss of fistula
Thromboses	67 (69%)	37 (55%)	30 (45%)
Stenoses	13 (14%)	9 (69%)	4 (45%)
Hematoma	3 (3%)	3 (100%)	–
Infections	7 (7%)	1 (14%)	6 (86%)
Aneurysm	7 (7%)	4 (57%)	3 (43%)
n	97 (100%)	54 (55%)	43 (45%)

Thromboses and stenoses were more frequent in Cimino fistula than in Goretex fistula (55 % vs 31 % and 62 % vs 7 %, resp.) Infections were only observed in Goretex fistula. Stenoses and thromboses were observed earlier in homologous venous transplants (mean interval five months) than in Cimino- (mean interval 41 months) or in Goretex fistula (mean interval 38 months).

Conclusion: In Cimino fistula, stenoses and thrombotic occlusions are the most frequent fistula complications leading to loss of the vascular access in 45 %. Infections are most frequent in prostheses resulting in loss of the vascular access in almost all fistulae. In search for alternative therapy, homologous venous transplants have a high incidence of early stenoses and thromboses.

These data may have a clinical relevance with regard to prospective erythropoietin therapy.

Hickman Catheters as a Long-Term Vascular Access for Hemodialysis in Adult Patients

J. DE MEESTER, R. VANHOLDER, S. RINGOIR

Abstract

Between December 1985 and December 1987, 18 Hickman catheters were inserted in 14 patients in a subclavian or a deep jugular position, as a continuous vascular access for hemodialysis. In all patients, all other access possibilities had been exhausted. Five patients had been withdrawn from CAPD because of repeated peritonitis and/or ultrafiltration problems. In three other patients, CAPD was considered to be impossible because of repeated abdominal interventions. The mean age of these patients was 56.8 ± 20.2 years. Nine patients were older than 50 and six were older than 65 years. The duration of previous renal replacement therapy averaged 56.1 ± 61.0 months. Five patients had a follow-up of more than 60 months (89 to 182 months). Follow-up data are available up to June 1988. Catheters remained in place for a mean period of 192.6 ± 200.2 days. In the seven patients that maintained a viable catheter at the end of the follow-up period, follow-up averaged 386.0 ± 197.6 days (range 217 to 610 days). Two fatalities occurred that were not related to the Hickman catheter. The most frequent complication was inadequate flow (n = 10), either with or without clotting (n = 5 each). This problem was resolved by Fogarty catheterization (n = 2) or the introduction of a new catheter (n = 4), but resulted in the failure of the technique in four cases. No infections occurred. Technique failure was significantly more frequent in catheters without side holes (cumulative survival after five months: 37 %), compared to catheters with one or two side holes (86 %). Dialysis efficiency appeared to be good. In conclusion, Hickman catheterization appears to be a valuable alternative vascular access, especially in elderly patients where other access methods have been exhausted. Inadequate flow remains a major problem, especially in catheters without side holes.

Introduction

Hemodialysis made it possible to maintain uremic patients alive, and to improve their life quality. For this blood purification technique access to the vascular bed is a must; vascular access remains however the Achilles heel of modern dialysis. In the early days of dialysis, access was obtained by arterial and venous puncture or catheterization. Chronic maintenance hemodialysis on a large scale became only possible after the introduction of the arterio-venous shunt by Scribner [1] but this access system continues to have numerous problems. Long term dialysis without major pitfalls was enabled by the development of the arterio-venous fistula by Cimino and Brescia in 1966 [2]. Maturation of a Cimino-Brescia fistula however necessitates a waiting time of three to 8 weeks. Therefore, this method is not suitable for acute situations, where a quick access is needed. Central venous catheterization offers this possibility. The three most obvious insertion sites are the subclavian, deep jugular and femoral veins.

Nevertheless, there remain multiple problems with central vein catheterization for hemodialysis. First, the blind introduction of catheters via needle puncture may cause a number of traumatic complications [3-6]; these complications are observed only rarely but may have dramatic consequences; especially with catheters in the subclavian and the femoral position. A number of fatalities due to hemothorax and hemoperitoneum, have been described [7, 8]. A second problem is that some trivial complications, like infection and inadequate flow occur rather frequently, and may affect the patients condition and the adequacy of dialysis [3]. The latter problems are related to the biocompatibility of dialysis catheters for central venous use.

All these problems have resulted in the use of central vein catheters for only limited periods of time. Long term use may result in subclavian vein or superior caval vein thrombosis or occlusion [9, 10]. Nevertheless, it may be necessary to use the central venous access way for longer periods of time, especially if it is difficult or impossible to use alternative solutions.

A few years ago, Hickman catheters were propagated as an alternative access method for prolonged use in infants [11]. In view of the frequent access problems in adults, especially in the elderly and in patients who have been dialyzed for prolonged periods of time, this access method was used in our unit, as a last resource, since December 1985. This paper summarizes our experience in this field.

Materials and Methods

A follow-up study was conducted from December 1985 on. All catheters inserted up to December 1987 were studied. The follow-up study was terminated the first of June 1988. All patients were stable chronic dialysis patients and they were treated 3-4 hours weekly with a single needle method and on bicarbonate dialysate. Catheters were only inserted via a surgical technique. Flexible silicone rubber catheters with a length of 15 to 26 cm were used. Care was taken to position the catheter tip in the superior vena cava, and an atrial position was avoided. Control of the position was performed by radioscopy during the surgical introduction, and absence of resistance was checked by abrupt aspiration of blood from the catheter. The proximal part of the catheter was positioned in a subcutaneous tunnel.

The catheter is surrounded by a cuff that is positioned in the subcutaneous tunnel near to the skin exit site to protect the tunnel from entry of bacteria.

Catheters were either positioned in a jugular or a subclavian position. Jugular catheterization was preferred, unless the latter procedure was impossible, or unless problems were expected, as patients had a history of repeated jugular catheterization or neck region surgery in their antecedents. No side holes, or one or two side holes were created near the catheter tip on a random basis. The side holes were positioned at five mm of the catheter tip. In one case, more than two side holes were created.

Catheters were used for dialysis within 24 hours after the insertion. After use, they were filled with 1.25 ml of heparin, until the next use. In most patients, ticlopidine was administered p.o. to avoid clotting at the catheter tip. Skin sterilization and change of dressings were performed as indicated.

For each of the patients under study, the previous history, the reasons for the use of a Hickman catheter, eventual complications, and the period over which the catheter remained viable were registered. Furthermore, in a number of patients, data on efficiency of dialysis were registered at regular intervals, as previously described [12].

Results

Between December 1985 and December 1987, Hickman catheters were inserted in 14 patients. Seven were males and seven females. Their mean age was 56 years (range 11 to 81 years). Nine patients were older than 50 years, and six patients were older than 65 years. In all patients, all other access possibilities had been exhausted. Five of these patients had previously been withdrawn from CAPD because of repeated peritonitis and/or ultrafiltration problems. In three other patients, CAPD was considered to be impossible because of repeated abdominal interventions.

Five patients had previously not been treated by hemodialysis. In the remaining nine patients, hemodialysis had been performed before the Hickman catheterization over a mean period of time of 54 months.

Three patients had previously not been treated by any form of renal replacement therapy. In the remaining 11 patients the total treatment time (hemodialysis and/or CAPD and/or transplantation), averaged 64 months (range 8 to 77 months).

Four patients had been treated with more than one technique before the start of Hickman catheter dialysis: hemodialysis and CAPD in 3, hemodialysis, CAPD and transplantation in one patient.

As noted in Table 1, a total number of 18 catheters was inserted. Eleven patients received only one catheter, two patients received two catheters and one patient received three catheters. Subsequently, eight catheter failures were noticed, but in four cases the technique could be continued with another catheter. The four

Table 1. Catheters.

n = 18	Technique failure	Transition to
11 patients : 1 catheter 2 patients : 2 catheters 1 patient : 3 catheters	catheter failures = 8 access failures = 4	CAPD 2 × intermittent femoral catheterization 1 × conservative treatment 1 ×

technique failures were observed in two patients who had received only one catheter, whereas one of these patients received two and another three catheters. Two patients were transferred to CAPD, one to intermittent femoral catheterization, and one to conservative treatment. Two patients died for reasons not related to the Hickman technique. The relation between the number of sideholes and failure rate is illustrated in Table 2. Catheters without side holes showed a failure rate of 60 %. Catheters with one and two side holes together had a failure rate of only 14 % (33 and 0 % respectively). The single catheter with more than two side holes failed. Cumulative survival after five months was only 37 % for catheters without sideholes, compared to 86 % for catheters with one or two sideholes ($p < 0.05$).

Table 2. Relation between number of sideholes and failure rate.

Number of Sideholes	Number of Catheters	Failures	Percentage
0	10	6	60
1	3	1	33
2	4	0	0
> 2	1	1	100

Catheters remained in place for a mean period of 192.6 ± 200.2 days. In the seven patients that maintained a viable catheter at the end of the follow-up period, follow-up averaged 386.0 ± 197.6 (range 217-610 days).

The most frequently observed problem (Table 3) was certainly the occurence of inadequate flow. This was due to clotting in five cases. Two of these problems could be resolved by Fogarty catheterization. Two patients received a new catheter, and in one patient the technique was stopped. Of five cases without clotting, two patients received a new catheter, and in three the technique was stopped. Attempts to use streptokinase ($n = 3$) did not result in declotting. In two patients, streptokinase was not used because of their age. It should be stressed that most of the flow problems occurred in catheters without side holes ($n = 6$) and/or were registered repeatedly in one patient (one patient with two and one patient with three episodes respectively).

If expressed per days of follow-up, this occurrence of flow problems is still lower than that observed with intermittent subclavian and internal jugular catheters (2.9 cases per 1000 days of follow-up for Hickman catheters vs 3.8 for subclavian and jugular catheters). If this type of calculation is restricted to Hickman catheters with one or two sideholes, occurrence is 1.7/1000.

Table 3. Complications.

Flow Problems	Number		
With Clotting	5	Fogarty New Catheter Stop Technique	2 2 1
Without Clotting	5	New Catheter Stop Technique	2 3
Bleeding (Local)	4		
Infection	0		

The occurrence of 0 infections for 3467 days of follow-up should be compared to an incidence of 3.0/1000 for classical intermittent catheters.

Dialysis adequacy was estimated in a limited number of cases (Table 4). Blood flow (Q_B), urea and creatinine dialyzer clearance (K_D), recirculation (R), and dialyzer clearance corrected for recirculation (K_C), all appeared to be efficient, and not subjected to variations.

Discussion

In this paper, our experience concerning the continuous use of Hickman catheters in central venous position is reported. Hickman catheters have previously been described as efficient for the administration of parenteral nutrition and anti-cancer treatment [13, 14]. After an adaptation for the large flows created in hemodialysis, Hickman catheters were also used for the latter technique in children [11].

Table 4. Dialysis Efficiency Data.

	1 Month (n = 4)	3 Months (n = 4)	6 Months (n = 4)	Overall (n = 4)
Q_B (ml/min)	241.3 ± 59.8	280.6 ± 76.5	268.4 ± 46.1	266.4 ± 56.6
K_D (ml/min)				
Urea	148.1 ± 12.2	167.8 ± 15.8	158.3 ± 5.0	158.1 ± 13.7
Creatinine	123.8 ± 8.7	135.4 ± 11.9	127.2 ± 3.1	128.8 ± 9.2
R (%)				
Urea	14.5 ± 10.0	17.8 ± 8.1	13.0 ± 7.1	15.1 ± 7.9
Creatinine	13.5 ± 9.0	20.4 ± 6.4	17.6 ± 5.6	16.9 ± 7.1
K_C (ml/min)				
Urea	136.7 ± 10.9	145.8 ± 12.9	145.4 ± 3.6	142.6 ± 10.0
Creatinine	116.7 ± 13.2	125.7 ± 10.1	113.9 ± 9.7	118.8 ± 11.4

Data obtained 1, 3 and 6 months after catheter insertion.
Overall: mean of all values together.

Cases of catheters positioned in adults in a central vein or the right atrium are also reported [15, 16]. Our present experience on 18 catheters shows that this treatment type can offer adequate dialysis and an alternative access possibility, especially in those patients where other treatment and access modalities have been exhausted. A substantial number of the patients reported here had a long and complicated history of renal replacement therapy (in one patient more than 15 years). In many of them CAPD was impossible or undesirable. A substantial fraction was older than 65.

The main problem with this catheter technique is certainly the presence of flow problems, however this is largely restricted to catheters without side holes and with a tendency to recur in the same patients. If occurence is expressed per days of follow-up, frequency is lower than with the more current intermittent central vein catheterization techniques. Other complications are trivial. The risk of infection is virtually nil.

Most flow problems appear to occur shortly after the insertion of the catheter. Once this period is over, the risk of this complication becomes extremely low, and dialysis is efficient and stable. Eventual problems can in some case be treated by a Fogarty technique. The use of streptokinase is not successful. Ticlopidine may be administered to prevent clotting problems.

In conclusion, central vein hemodialysis via Hickman catheters appears to be a valuable alternative access method, especially in those patients with a long history of renal replacement therapy, where adequate access possibilities are lacking, and in the elderly. The complication profile is low, and the main complication, flow problems, may largely be prevented by the use of catheters with one or two sideholes, and the preventive administration of ticlopidine.

References

[1] Quinton, W. E., D. Dillard, B. H. Scribner: Cannulation of blood vessels for prolonged hemodialysis. *Trans. Am. Soc. Artif. Organs* 6: 104-113 (1960).

[2] Brescia, M. J., J. E. Cimino, K. Appel, B. J. Hurwich: Chronic hemodialysis using venipuncture and a surgically created venous fistula. *New Engl. J. Med.* 275: 1089-1092 (1966).

[3] Vanholder, R., N. A. Hoenich, S. Ringoir: Morbidity and mortality of central venous hemodialysis: a review of 10 years' experience. *Nephron* 47: 274-279 (1987).

[4] Bambauer, R., G. A. Jutzler: Erfahrungen mit grosslumigen Verweilkathetern in der V. jugularis interna als Zugang für akute Hämodialysen. *Klin. Wochenschr.* 60: 285-292 (1982).

[5] Shaldon, S., L. Chiandussi, B. Higgs: Haemodialysis by percutaneous catheterization of the femoral artery and vein with regional heparinisation. *Lancet* 2: 857-859 (1961).

[6] Vanholder, R. C., S. Ringoir: Percutaneous femoral vessel cannulation for hemodialysis, pp. 129-152. In: Andreucci, V. E. (ed.): Vascular and peritoneal access for dialysis. Kleuver Academic Publ., Boston 1989.

[7] Kjellstrand, C., G. E. Merino, S. M. Mauer, R. Casali, T. J. Buselmeier: Complications of percutaneous femoral vein catheterizations for hemodialysis. *Clin. Nephrol.* 4: 37-40 (1975).

[8] Uldall, P. R.: Subclavian cannulation for hemodialysis: the present state of the art. *Artif. Organs* 6: 73-76 (1982).

[9] VAN HERWEGHEM, J. L., T. YASSINE, M. GOLDMAN, G. VANDENBOSCH, C. DELCOUR, J. STRUYEN, P. KINNAERT: Subclavian vein thrombosis: a frequent complication of subclavian vein cannulation for hemodialysis. *Clin. Nephrol.* 26: 235-238 (1986).

[10] VANHOLDER, R., N. LAMEIRE, J. VERBANCK, R. VAN RATTINGHE, M. KUNNEN, S. RINGOIR: Complications of subclavian catheter hemodialysis: a 5-year prospective study in 257 consecutive patients. *Int. J. Artif. Organs* 5: 297-303 (1982).

[11] SCHROEDER, P., T. CHANG, R. ENGEMANN, P. JESSEN, W. MENGEL: Der Hickman-Katheter als permanenter Zugang zur Hämodialyse beim Kind. *Chirurg* 58: 179-181 (1987).

[12] VANHOLDER, R., N. A. HOENICH, S. RINGOIR: Dialysis performance of single lumen subclavian hemodialysis: a comparative study with single lumen fistula hemodialysis. *Artif. Organs* 6: 429-432, (1982).

[13] RIELLA, M. C., B. H. SCRIBNER: Five years experience with a right atrial catheter for prolonged parenteral nutrition at home. *Surg. Gyn. Obstet.* 143: 205-208 (1976).

[14] HICKMAN, R., C. D. BUCKNER, R. A. CLIFT, J. E. SANDERS, P. STEWART, E. D. THOMAS: A modified right atrial catheter for access to the venous system in marrow transplant recipients. *Surg. Gyn. Obstet.* 148: 871-875 (1979).

[15] FRANCIS, D. M. A., N. A. HOENICH, R. M. R. TAYLOR, M. K. WARD, D. N. S. KERR: An indwelling right atrial catheter for long-term hemodialysis. *Trans. Am. Soc. Artif. Int. Organs* 29: 348-351 (1983).

[16] FRANCIS, D. M. A., M. K. WARD, R. M. R. TAYLOR: Right-atrial catheters for long-term vascular access in haemodialysis patients. *Lancet* 2: 301-302 (1982).

Our Eight Years Experience with Subclavian Catheters for Hemodialysis

J. VARL, J. DRINOVEC, A. GUČEK, R. PONIKVAR, R. KVEDER

Abstract

Experience with 555 subclavian dialysis catheters in the period from 1980 to 1988 was reviewed. The catheters were placed in 385 patients and were inserted 17.6 ±14 days. The longest placement was more than one year. There were immediate serious complications in 0.6 %. Unsuccessful cannulation occured in 7.5 %, puncture of subclavian artery in 2.5 %. Removal of the catheter due to local or/and systemic infection occured in 11.9 %, occlusion of the catheter in 12.2 %. 323 catheters remained inserted with tunnelisation.

Introduction

The adequate vascular approach for acute hemodialysis treatment represents always a specific problem. Percutaneous subclavian venous cannulation allows immediate and safe enough access to the vascular bed for hemodialysis. The quick and relative ease of insertion, mobility of patient, length of use and avoidance of new potential access sites contributes to this method's popularity in recent years [1-4].

Looking for this, our experience with subclavian catheters for hemodialysis in patients with acute renal failure or chronic renal failure is given.

Patients and Methods

A follow up study was conducted in the period from January 1980 to March 1988. In this period 555 subclavian dialysis catheters were placed in 385 patients. The age of patients was 46 ±16 years (range 5-85 years). There were two groups of patients: the group with acute renal failure and the group with chronic renal failure with (a) rapid deterioration of renal failure or (b) thrombosis of A-V fistula.

The subclavian catheters (made of polyurethane or teflon) were introduced according to the Seldinger technique. 323 catheters were inserted with tunnelisation, while 232 catheters were placed without it. We started with tunnelisation in April 1983. Chest radiographs were obtained in all patients to document the position of the catheter. To maintain patency of the catheters they were flushed with saline and filled with heparin.

Results

The catheters remained in place 17.6 $\pm$14 days (range 1-368 days). The duration of insertion of the catheters was as follows: 1-7 days in 25 %, 8-14 days in 24.7 %, 15-30 days in 33.4 %, 31-60 days in 15.4 % and more than 60 days in 1.4 %. In one patient the subclavian catheter remained in place for more than one year (368 days). Complications were divided as follows:

a) immediate serious complications and

b) complications related to insertion itself.

Looking at group (a) they occured in 0.9 % (two hemothoraxes, one pneumothorax, one mediastinal hematoma and one lesion of trachea with hemoptysis). Complications by insertion of the catheter were as follows: unsuccessful cannulation in 7.5 %, puncture of subclavian artery in 2.5 % and difficult insertion in 7.1 %.

There were several causes of removal of the catheters: infection (local or systemic) in 11.9 %, avulsion in 6.5 %, occlusion of the catheter in 12.2 %. The catheters were removed in 10.4 % because restoration of kidney function took place, in 19 % a new A-V fistula was constructed. Death occured in 36 severely ill patients, 72 patients were transported with functioning subclavian catheters to other hospitals and were lost for the follow up.

Discussion

Insertion of subclavian dialysis catheter is well established vascular access in patients with acute or chronic renal failure. This catheters can be rapidly introduced, give adequate blood flow for dialysis and can be left in place for several days or weeks. In our study the majority of the catheters remained inserted between two and four weeks (33.4 %). Complications related to cannulation of the vessels were low and none was life threatening. The percentage of complications in our study remarkably was higher at the beginning when the method was introduced. Death occured in 36 severy ill patients but none was directly related to the insertion of the subclavian catheter. Infection (local or systemic) was one of the most important complications and the catheter withdrawal was necessary in almost 12 %. Insertion with tunnelisation diminishes the mechanical complications due to handling of the catheter during hemodialysis but has no major influence on diminishing the frequency of infection.

Conclusions

On the basis of our data we can conclude that insertion of a subclavian catheter for hemodialysis is safe enough for urgent vascular access. It requires some experience, rigid aseptic conditions and careful follow up. Although a subclavian catheter offers many advantages including quick placement, patient mobility and preservation of peripheral blood vessels for future access, infection remains the most serious complication for the patient.

References

[1] VANHOLDER, R., N. A. HOENICH, S. RINGOIR: Morbidity and Mortality of Central Venous Catheter Hemodialysis: A Review of 10 Year's Experience. *Nephron* 47: 274-279 (1987).

[2] CHEESBROUGH, J. S., R. G. FINCH, R. P. BURDEN: A Prospective Study of the Mechanisms of Infection Associated with Hemodialysis Catheters. *J. Infect. Dis.* 154: 579-589 (1986).

[3] ERBEN, J., J. KVASNICKA, J. BASTECKY: Long-term Experience with the Technique of Subclavian and femoral Vein Cannulation in Hemodialysis. *Art. Organs* 3: 241-244 (1979).

[4] DAHLBERG, P. J., W. R. YUTUC, K. L. NEWCOMER: Subclavian Hemodialysis Catheter Infections. *Am. J. Kidney Dis.* 7: 421-427 (1986).

Red Cell Fragmentation Syndrome in Chronic Single Needle Dialysis

R. HOMBROUCKX, A. M. BOGAERT, F. LEROY, L. LARNO, J. Y. DE VOS

Abstract

Hemolysis is an underestimated phenomen in single needle dialysis. A prospective study was started in 1985 in 30 stable chronic patients. During 10,000 single needle dialysis sessions hemolysis was systematically screened. We selected the rise in serum lactic dehydrogenase (LDH) as a parameter for hemolysis. We found some degree in hemolysis in most patients during every dialysis, but with increasing degree of hemolysis we noted symptoms as nausea, headache, vomitus, epigastric pain, retrosternal oppression, hypotension without shock but lasting for one or two days, dyspnoe, flushing, cyanosis of lips and nailbeds, oesophagal spasms, angina pectoris or abdominis, resistant to nitrates and oxygen, lumbar pains, subicterus, severe abdominal or retrosternal pain, shock, icterus and arrythmias.

The biological stigmata were a raised serum LDH, bilirubin and reticulocytosis, a macrocytosis (by the preferential destruction of older RBC), anemia, and a low or absent serum haptoglobin. The longterm effects are anemia and iron overload.

Different combinations of peripheral needle and central catheter dialysis enabled us to localize the site of the hemolysis: namely the tip of the peripheral needle by a too high shear stress.

Introduction

Since the last decade there was a trend towards a decrease in dialysis duration (by increasing the blood flow) and towards single needle techniques – two strategies that negatively could influence the red blood cell (RBC) integrity. We systematically screened for two years the mechanical destruction of RBC on red cell fragmentation (RCF) during each dialysis session on the double head pump (DHP) unipuncture system in 30 chronic stabilized patients.

Other causes of intravascular hemolysis (HL) than the mechanical destruction of RBC have been ruled out (e.g. serological factors, hemoglobinopathies, RBC-membrane defects, enzymatic deficiencies, micro-angiopathic factors, infectious agents, drug induced hemolysis, etc.).

Material and Methods

After an initial period of broad screening for HL, we selected as a practical hemolysis index (HLI) the increase of lactic acid dehydrogenase (LDH) in the serum during dialysis.

$$\text{HLI} = \frac{\text{LDH serum level postdialysis}}{\text{LDH serum level predialysis}}$$

Care must be taken for artificial HL during blood sample taking and laboratory processing.

Results

It appeared that the HLI per patient remained practically unchanged over several dialyses, in other words, the HLI was more or less a constant factor per patient (Fig. 1); only a few patients showed a HLI of one (=no HL).

Type of HL:

1. A broad hematological screening showed no differences between severe and less hemolytic patients (no known genetic or acquired factors could be shown as responsible for differences in HLI between patients).
   We had to conclude for mechanical RCF by exclusion of other causes of HL and by the appearance of fragmentocytes or schistocytes.
2. We also tried to influence the degree of HL by adding O_2, Vit. C, glucose and ATP (pure or in combinations) to the dialysate, but this proved unsuccessful. A very limited benefit was encountered for Vit. E as chronic p.o. medication, no significant effect was seen for Cinnarizine.
3. We also looked for the site of HL in the SND: the observation that in central catheter SND no demonstrable RCF occured excluded blood-lines, expansion chamber, artificial kidney and pump segments as RCF factor.

Different combinations of two needle dialysis by means of a central catheter plus a peripheral catheter needle proved the peripheral catheter needle to be the factor responsible for RCF.

Further tests enabled us to localize the RCF in the needle tip. New experimental anti-hemolytic needle or peripheral catheter types are being tested now with very good results.

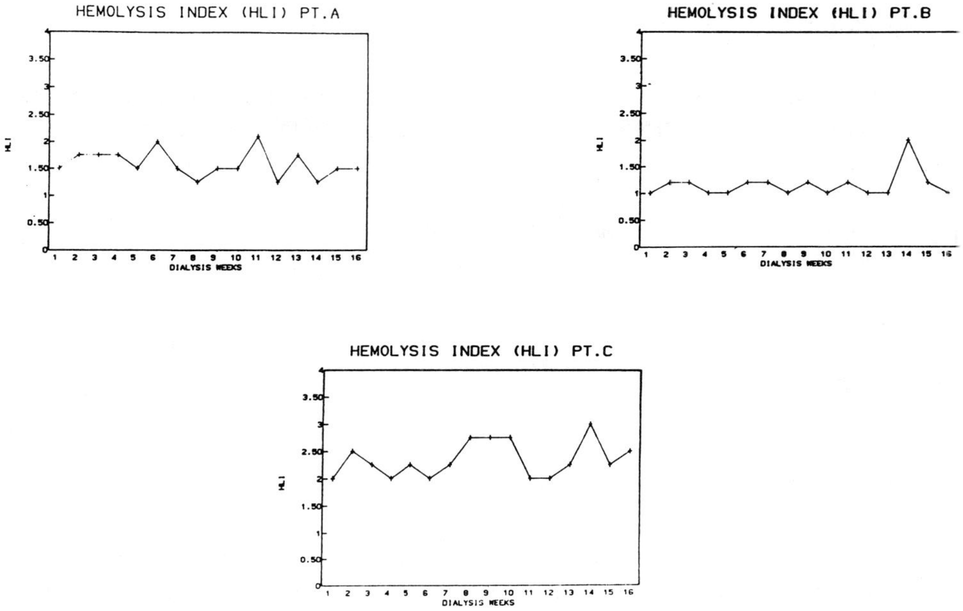

Fig. 1. Hemolysis Index for three patients.

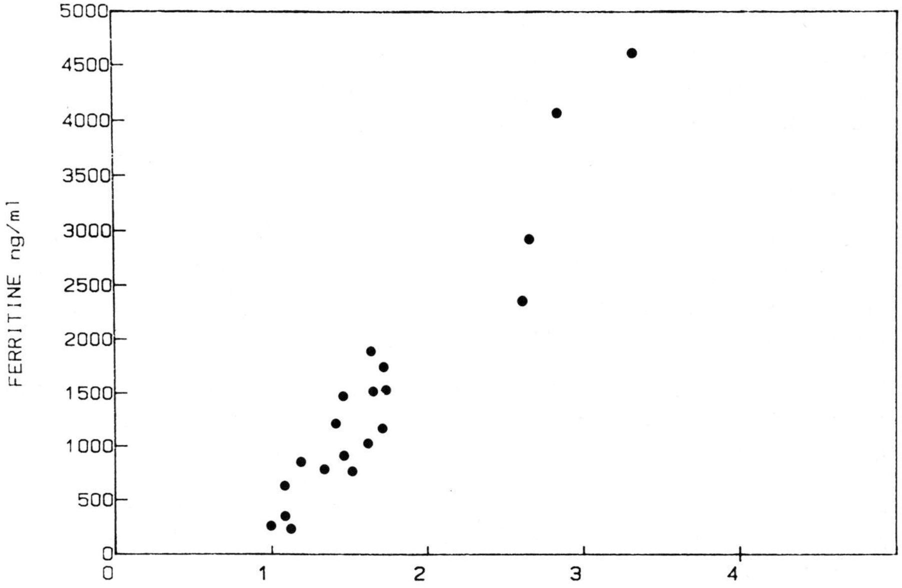

Fig. 2. Patients more than five years on dialysis.

Discussion

1. The symptoms during the dialysis session attributed to RCF were, with increasing degree of HL: nervousness, anxiety, epigastric malaise, nausea, headache, epigastric or retrosternal pain, vomitus, hypotension, cyanosis of lips and nailbeds, oesophagal spasms after dialysis, interdialytic hypotension, flushing, angina, shock, cyanosis, icterus.
   For each degree of HLI there were the corresponding symptoms.
2. We noted the coincidence of several parameters, namely the predialysis level of LDH and bilirubin, a macrocytosis and a reticulocytosis, but also a severe hyperferritinemia in high grade HLI patients – (in contrast to RCF in normal individuals, there is an important iron overload in hemolytic dialysis patients; Fig. 2); this was proven by a liver biopsy in several patients. Previously unexplained liver test disturbances and splenomegalies proved to be due to chronic RCF, and disappeared after HL reduction.

Conclusion

1. The site of the RCF was not, as previously accepted, the pump segments of the roller blood pump, but the needle tip. Newer experimental needle types give a significantly lower degree of HL for blood flows up to 250 ml/min.
2. This Chronic RCF on SND is an important clinical problem, until now for the most part unknown and underestimated.
3. We have to think about RCF in cases of:
   - bad dialysis tolerance (hypotension, nausea, anxiety), recurrent angina or even infarction symptoms during dialysis; interdialytic hypotension or oesophagal spasms;
   - anemia, reticulocytosis, macrocytosis, hyperbilirubinemia;
   - iron overload, unexplained liver test disturbances (pseudo-non A- non B-hepatitis) and splenomegaly, especially in chronic single needle dialysis on peripheral needles or catheter needles.

Bidirectional Blood-Pump with a Bidirectional Blood-Passage through the Artificial Kidney

R. HOMBROUCKX, R. BEELEN, A. M. BOGAERT, F. LEROY, J. Y. DE VOS

Abstract

A new single needle dialysis system was developed, inspired on the highly efficient pigeons' respiratory system: a double passage through the exchange organ was envisaged. We therefore tested a bidirectional roller pump that first lifts the blood through the unique needle, the unique bloodline and the artificial kidney, fills up an accumulation bag placed above the artificial kidney (first passage), and then switches direction at a preselected maximum weight in the accumulation bag and empties this bag through the artificial kidney again (second passage). The pump is thus directed by a minimum and maximum weight setting.

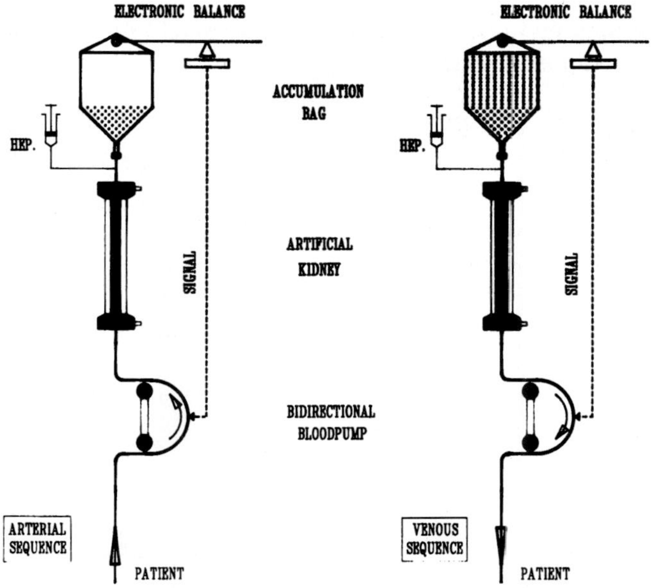

Fig. 1. Bidirectional blood pump.

The main disadvantage of the system is some amount of recirculation of non-filtered blood, namely the content of bloodline, pump segment and lower part of the artificial kidney; for this reason the bloodpump has to be kept as small as possible.

However this recirculation or "ineffective blood flow" is overcompensated by the "effective blood flow".

The system is very simple (can be applied by a patient alone without partner), is very cheap, has a low bloodpriming and permits a perfect ultrafiltration control. Already 1000 dialysis are performed over two years in six patients with the experimental prototypes.

Introduction

Inspired by the very efficient respiratory system of the pigeon, a new single-needle dialysis system has been developed, whereby a double passage of the blood through the exchange organ (this being the artificial kidney – AK) was contemplated.

We tested a bidirectional blood-pump (BDP; Fig. 1), which through one needle and one blood line pumps the blood from the blood vessel then guides it through the AK (first passage; Fig. 2) to an accumulation bag (AB), located above the AK; the weight of that bag is monitored and upon attaining a preset max. weight, the pump changes direction, empties the exp. bag through the AK (second passage; Fig. 3) and directs the blood back into the patient's blood vessel. The pump is controlled by a min. and max. weight setting, the weight of the accumulation bag being recorded by an electronic balance.

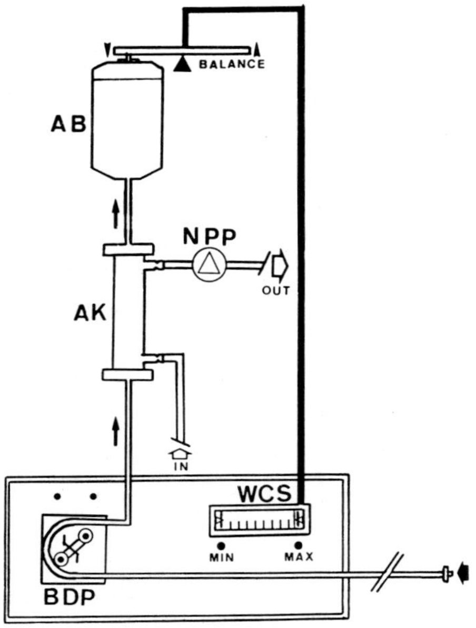

Fig. 2. First passage.

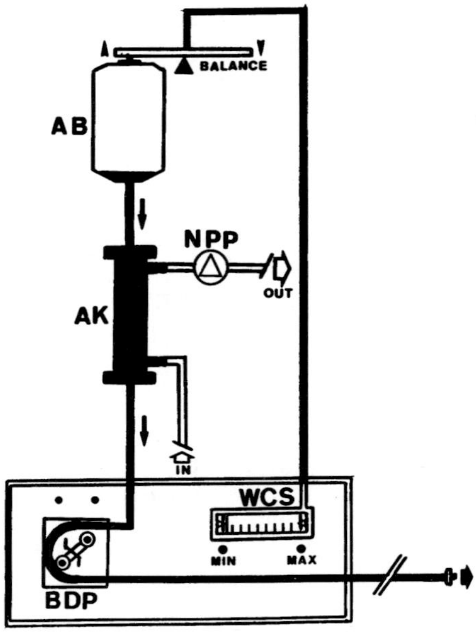

Fig. 3. Second passage.

Equipments and Methods

The system consists of one bipuncture needle, a modified blood line, the bidirectional blood pump (BDP), this being a compact peristaltic blood pump, modified for bidirectional functioning by us. Further, there is the artificial kidney that may be of any type, on condition that it has a low blood priming volume, a low dialysate priming volume and a rigid membrane structure (thus for preference a capillary kidney). There also is the accumulation bag (AB), which consists in a flaccid plastic bag (e.g. Flex Flac or Viaflex) with a maximum content of 500 ml; this bag is connected through a small blood line to the artificial kidney. The bag is suspended on the arm of an electronic balance.

The bidirectional blood-pump is controlled by way of min. and max. weight setting.

The ultrafiltration is monitored through the dialysate side (ultrafiltration pump on controled ultrafiltration).

Functioning

1. *Patient's blood flow*
   = the stroke volume × the frequency of the cycle.

$$= \frac{\text{Stroke volume} \times 60}{\text{Arterial + venous cycle in seconds}}.$$

2. *Effective patient's blood flow*
   = patient's blood flow reduced by the dead volume (being the capacity of the blood lines, pump segments and the lower part of artificial kidney)
   = (stroke volume − dead volume) × frequency.

3. *Artificial kidney blood flow*
   = twice the patient's blood flow reduced by the recirculating volume or dead volume

$$= \frac{(\text{Stroke volume} - \text{dead volume}) \times 60 \times 2}{\text{Arterial + venous cycle in seconds}}.$$

Safeties

- Air and foam-microdetector in blood line between needle and pump head (pump stop plus visible and audible alarm).
- Low-pressure detection between needle and pump head.

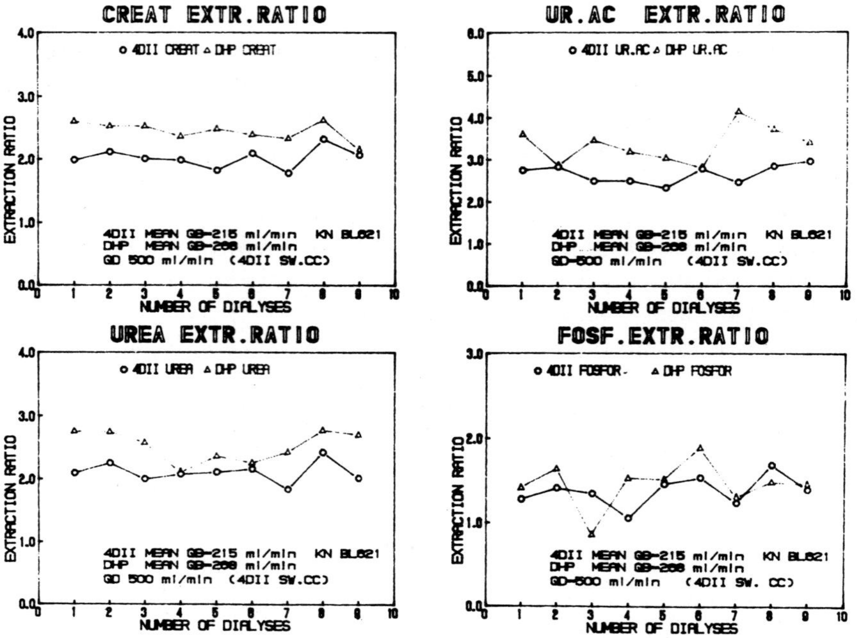

Fig. 4. Extraction ratios.

- (Excess-pressure detection between pump head and needle.)
- Incorporated revolution-counter in the pump (in the event of excessive pump head rotation the pump stops and a visual and audible alarm is given).
- Cumulative counter of the number of venous pump head rotations (measuring the cumulative blood flow through the system).

Results

The overall dialysis ratios for most molecules are comparable with the double headpump (DHP) results (Fig. 4); however, the bidirectional AK passage results in a better extraction pattern for phosphate, especially when the direction of the dialysate flow is changed (Fig. 5).

$$\text{Dialysis ratio} = \frac{\text{patient's serum concentration before dialysis}}{\text{patient's serum concentration after dialysis}}$$

Discussion

The greatest disadvantage of the system is the recirculation of the dead volume blood (content of blood line and pump segment) which reduces the overall efficiency of the system. However, as soon as the stroke volume becomes three to four times greater than the dead volume, this recirculation has an almost negligible effect on the ultimate efficiency. To avoid excessive stroke volumes, we naturally miniaturize the system as much as possible. The ultrafiltration control is obtained by negative pressure setting in the dialysate compartment (ultrafiltration pump). It is the only single needle system wherein the high peak flows that pass through the needle, also effectively pass through the kidney and this in both directions per cycle.

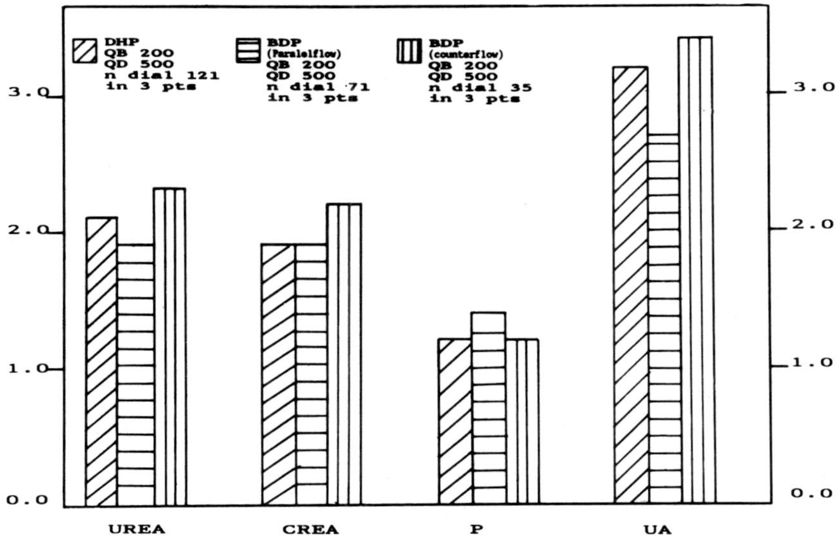

Fig. 5. Dialysis ratio DR = (Pre) / (Post).

Conclusion

1. Simple system, which renders it suitable for home- and low-care dialysis (can be carried out by a patient without a partner), but just as suitable for routine dialysis or hemofiltration.
2. The high effective bidirectional flow through the artificial kidney renders the system, according to the direction of the dialysate flow, suitable for a more selective clearing of either small molecules or of phosphorus and middle molecules.

3. There is no risk for air-embolism: even if the accumulation bag is empty, no air enters the system; the pump will be stopped by foam alarm, by the counter control or by underpressure alarm.
4. Low priming volume, which reduces periods of hypotension during the dialysis and which also makes a rinse-back with a minimal quantity of saline possible.
5. The system fits into the dialysis strategy of daily ultrashort dialysis to be carried out by the patient himself (without partner – either at home, or in a collective auto-dialysis centre).
6. Very economical system, as concerns both the disposables and the hardware.
7. By the lower number of pump head switchings, also less hemolysis than in other tidal single needle systems.

Permanent Vascular Access: Long-Term Results

A. STALTERI, G. LO PICCOLO, F. MONTELEONE, F. DI GIOVANNA

Abstract

This paper summarizes the 90 months access surgery at Sciacca Hospital, Italy. The high overall patency rate of A-V fistulas contrast with very poor results in systemic vasculopathic patients. The goal of prolonged access survival can be achieved by correct planning of the use of upper limb superficial vessels, whenever possible. The authors report two cases of steal and four cases of flow velocity reduction of vertebral artery, induced by homolateral proximal A-V fistula: a new dialysis side effect?

Introduction

Correct planning of the vascular access may become the chief factor in prolonged survival of patients with ESRD on renal replacement therapy (RRT). Wide use of external A-V shunts as acute temporary vascular access, and repeated attempts of secondary vascular access without a preliminary study of arterial and venous vessels of the forearm and arm, represent in our experience the main reasons of the Achilles heel [1] of the hemodialysis patients and of the increasing need of vascular prosthesis as permanent access.

This paper summarizes our clinical experience with the access surgery at Sciacca Hospital, a 500 bed-community hospital in Sciacca, Italy.

Patients and Methods

From December 1, 1980 to May 31, 1988, 160 uremic patients underwent 204 A-V fistulas (AVF) for hemodialysis. There were 82 females and 78 males; mean age was 58 years (range 14-85), mean dialytic age 62.5 months (range 2-183).

14 patients had adult-onset diabetes mellitus (AODM), three patients progressive systemic sclerosis (PSS) and two patients systemic lupus erythematosus (SLE) (19 patients with systemic vasculopathies = 11.9 %). Follow-up ranged from 2 to 90 months. AVF, under local anesthesia, were performed in upper limb, in distal site in 176 cases (82.2 %), or in proximal site in 28 cases (13.8 %).

Side-to-side (S-S) anastomosis were performed in 9.1 % of distal AVF, side-to-end (S-E) in 54.5 %, end-to-end (E-E) in 36.4 %. In four patients with failure of standard radio-cephalic fistula, side-to-side anastomosis was performed between the ulnar artery and the basilic vein of the forearm.

In 28 proximal AVF, the brachial artery was sutured to the cephalic (53.6 % of cases), or to the basilic vein (32.1 %), or to the basilic vein with side-to-end anastomosis and reverse flow (14.3 %).

In three patients with unsuitable peripheral vessels, A-V communications have been constructed utilising four Bio-Carbon transcutaneous hemodialysis access devices DiaTAB® (Amicon Bentley, Irvine, CA, USA).

For immediate treatment, up to September 1982, we implanted 24 Ramirez external A-V shunts (Johnson & Johnson, Anaheim, CA, USA); subsequently, for temporary vascular access, 128 femoral vein catheters (FC-100, Johnson & Johnson, Anaheim, CA, USA) were inserted in the groin using the Seldinger technique.

In all patients, before surgery for a secondary vascular access (AVF between the ulnar a. and the basilic v., proximal AVF, DiaTAB®) we performed venous angiography and continuous wave (CW) Doppler examination in order to map the route of specific vessels.

Prior to construction of proximal AVF, the last 20 consecutive patients were examined with CW Doppler, in order to evaluate the flow velocity on subclavian artery, common and internal carotid a., vertebral a. at ostium and Tillaux space.

We used a CW bidirectional velocity meter Doppler (Vasculab® mod. D-9, Meda-Sonics, Mountain View, CA, USA), with 4 and 8 MHz probes. For all operations, magnification loopes are regularly used. The survival curves were calculated by the life-table method [2].

Results

The overall patency rate (Table 1) was 75.5 % at 12 months, 69.5 % at two years, 64.9 % at five years; at the end of follow-up 64.1 % of AVF were patent. – The patency rate of angioaccess in systemic vasculopathic patients was 61.3 % at one year, 37.3 % at two years, 16.5 % at five years and 14.8 % at 90 months.

In 95 patients we performed only one vascular access, in 49 patients two operations; 11 patients were operated on three times and five patients needed four or more vascular access construction.

Ten early failures occurred within the first 48 hours; thrombosis, responsible for 100 % of these immediate failures, was due to hypotension and/or small size of the vessels and/or technical errors at operation.

36 AVF thrombosed ten days to 90 months after surgery: these late failures were due to prolonged hypotensive episode, large hematoma after needle cannulation, phlebitis, accidental trauma. In four cases we needed a second vascular access because of low-flow problems. In three patients we performed operative suppression of AVF (two cases developed venous hypertension – one patient had rupture of aneurysm of arterialized vein).

Table 1. Results of Angioaccess Patency Rate by Site and Type of Anastomosis. In the last column, results in 19 systemic vasculopathic patients.

Months	Total-AVF n = 204	D-AVF n = 176	D-AVF S-E	D-AVF E-E	D-AVF S-S	P-AVF n = 28	SVP-AVF n = 27
48 hr	95.8	96.7	96.0	96.9	96.4	96.4	95.4
1	90.1	90.3	90.4	90.2	90.0	89.1	92.5
6	81.1	81.2	81.0	82.3	81.0	81.3	86.9
12	75.5	80.5	80.8	80.3	80.3	76.9	61.3
24	69.5	78.3	77.1	79.2	79.1	73.3	37.3
36	67.2	73.2	74.0	73.6	73.0	70.5	27.5
48	66.5	70.7	70.0	71.0	71.0	66.2	26.9
60	64.9	68.4	69.2	67.5	66.9	62.8	16.5
90	64.1	65.6	65.2	65.8	65.6	58.7	14.8

D-AVF = Distal AVF; S-E = Side to end; E-E = End to end; S-S = Side to side; P-AVF = Proximal AVF; SVP = Systemic vasculopathic patients.

The patency rate of distal AVF was 80.5 % at one year, 78.3 % at two years, 68.4 % at five years; at the end of follow-up 65.6 % of distal AVF were patent.

We examined actuarial data on the survival of the three types of distal AVF (S-E, E-E, S-S), but there was no significant difference in the immediate failure rate or in the late failure rate.

The four S-S fistulas between the ulnar artery and the basilic vein of the forearm are patent with a mean patency rate of 20 months and a maximum function of 40 months. Two other ulnar-basilic fistulas stopped functioning within the first 48 hours.

The patency rate of 28 proximal AVF was 76.9 % at one year, 73.3 % at two years, 62.8 % at five years and 58.7 % at 90 months. These survival data are biased by disappointing results of the four reverse flow AVF: three patients with marked forearm edema – in two of them profound progressive swelling necessitated operative suppression of AVF one and eleven months after construction – in two other patients stasis and consequent thrombosis caused failure of reverse flow AVF 13 and 47 months after construction.

The first patient with PSS deceased two months after the DiaTAB® device was implanted from not related cause. Two DiaTAB® were implanted in a second patient with AODM: the first device stopped functioning after 12 months. The second device is patent after 20 months, but several episodes of fibrin flap formation under the plug were observed.

The third patient with AODM deceased 50 months after DiaTAB® implantation, from not related cause. These devices, in our experience, had a mean function time of 21 months and a maximum function time of 50 months. No problems were encountered with insertion of femoral catheters.

These catheters were left in situ 2-45 days (with a mean duration of 12.5 days). No major complications (hematoma, embolism, infections) were registered in our cases: in 22 % of patients we changed with a guide wire two or more femoral catheters because of low-flow problems, induced by the clotting of catheters bores.

The CW Doppler examination of 20 patients who underwent proximal AVF disclosed in two cases steal of vertebral artery, homolateral to AVF; in four cases there was a reduction of the flow velocity at the homolateral vertebral artery, induced by the Venturi effect.

Discussion

Maintenance of long-term angioaccess is the most challenging surgical effort performed for patients requiring chronic hemodialysis. For this purpose the essential thing is a correct planning of the use of upper limb superficial vessels in all patients who are potential candidates for RRT; these patients should be instructed not to let physicians or nurses use cephalic or antecubital veins for routine IV therapy or blood sampling. When dialysis is required, the first choice is S-E radio-cephalic fistula; this site can be used up to three times, if we avoid needling the first 4 cm of the arterialized cephalic vein.

The second choice is a fistula between the ulnar artery and the basilic vein of the forearm. The Allen test, performed by CW Doppler, offers assurance against ischemia of the hand.

The third choice is a proximal AVF between the distal brachial artery and the connecting branch to the cephalic vein at the antecubital fossa.

The fourth choice is to perform a brachio-basilic fistula, above the antecubital fossa.

Of course, we can utilize alternatively the two arms and then double our chances. The graft prosthesis should be utilized when superficial veins of the forearm and of the antecubital fossa will be exhausted. There are no data in our literature search about the steal or flow velocity reduction of the vertebral artery, induced by homolateral proximal AVF. This cranio-encephalic flow alteration may represent another dialysis side effect, but further wider investigations have to be made.

References

[1] Kjellstrand, C.: The Achilles' heel of the hemodialysis patient. *Arch. Int. Med.* 138: 1063-1064 (1978).

[2] Armitage, P., G. Berry (eds.): Statistical Methods in Medical Research. Blackwell: Oxford 1987.

Long-Term Experience with Hemodialysis Catheters Sepsis

M. Koselj, S. Kaplan, R. Ponikvar, A. Ličina, M. Gubina, J. Drinovec

Abstract

Since 1978 we have performed 2892 femoral vein dialysis catheters and 534 subclavian vein dialysis catheters. The femoral and the subclavian vein dialysis catheters were retrospectively evaluated for catheter-related sepsis. Femoral vein dialysis catheters have been in place for 7 to 67 days, subclavian vein dialysis catheters for 3 to 110 days. We found 38 culture proven cases of catheter-related sepsis in 35 patients. Femoral and subclavian vein dialysis catheters – tunneled – were associated with a low incidence of sepsis. S. aureus and S. epidermidis were the most common isolated microorganisms. These infections were easily managed with antibiotics and removal of the catheter.

Introduction

Percutaneous femoral or subclavian vein catheterization is a useful method for immediate but temporary access for hemodialysis.

Two complications limit the longevity of the dialysis catheter: clotting and infection. Infections of the access site are responsible for the majority of infections in patients on dialysis and are the source of 40 to 90 per cent of septicemic episodes [1]. The femoral vein is easier to cannulate but it does require that the patients be in the hospital if the catheter is left in place. The placement in this area is sufficiently benign that repeated introduction of the catheter is possible.

The subclavian site has the advantage of allowing the patient to ambulate. Because of the known tendency for infection in indwelling intravenous catheters, it is important to place and maintain the catheter in a strictly aseptic technique.

In an attempt to provide objective data regarding the quantity and risks of catheter-related sepsis, we have retrospectively reviewed the dialysis protocols of all adult patients at University Medical Center – Department of Nephrology Ljubljana, who had inserted femoral vein dialysis catheters (FVDCs) and subclavian vein dialysis catheters (SVDCs) in the last ten years.

Patients and Methods

From January 1978 through to December 1987 we have performed 2892 femoral vein cannulations and 534 subclavian vein cannulations.

The large vein catheters were placed in patients requiring hemodialysis for acute renal failure, and in patients with chronic renal failure who were awaiting vascular access or for the therapeutic plasma exchange.

Subclavian and femoral catheters were inserted by the renal unit medical staff. Francis catheter placement in the right atrium (a modification of Hickman's catheter) was done by vascular surgeon.

The insertion site was inspected prior to each dialysis and the dressing was changed after each dialysis. After initial insertion of the catheter, only dialysis nurses changed the dressing or manipulated the cannulas.

The catheter was used only for dialysis or plasma exchange.

If redness or purulent drainage was noted and when infection was suspected, cultures were taken from the drainage material and blood. If a positive blood culture was found and no other obvious source of sepsis was evident, the cannula was assumed to be the source and was immediately removed and appropriate antibiotics given. A new catheter can then be introduced on the opposite site.

Clinical evidence of catheter-related sepsis was considered by the growth of the same microorganisms from blood and catheter culture if the signs of sepsis resolved on its removal with antibiotics and if no alternative source of sepsis was revealed by clinical examination, chest radiograph or laboratory investigations.

The catheterization period was defined as the length of time the catheter occupied the same insertion site.

Results and Comment

During the period from January 1, 1978 through December 31, 1987, 3437 large vein cannulations were performed.

Femoral vein cannulation: 2892.

Subclavian vein cannulation: 534;

- tunneled: 261,
- nontunneled: 273.

Francis catheter in the right atrium: 11.

We found 38 septic complications (sepsis) among 35 patients with ARI or ESRD. Three of them were treated with plasma-exchange. Four patients had multisystemic disease. Four patients were diabetics.

There were 12 men and 23 women aged 17-79 years.

Femoral Catheters

Total 2892 femoral vein cannulations were used.
Number of sepsis: 14 or 0.48 %.
Blood culture: S. aureus, S. epidermidis, E. coli, Pseudomonas sp.
Catheterization period: 7-67 days, average 19.2 days.

Femoral catheters were inserted only for single use since January 1986 and septicemia due to catheter infection was not observed any more.

Subclavian Catheters

Total 534 subclavian vein cannulations were used
a) non-tunneled: 273;
catheterization period: 3-110 days, average 18.7 days,
number of sepsis: 16 or 5.9 %.
b) tunneled: 261;
catheterization period: 9-42 days, average 24.4 days,
number of sepsis: 5 or 1.9 %.
Blood culture: S. aureus, S. epidermidis, Proteus sp., Acinetobacter sp.

Francis Catheter in the Right Atrium

11 patients were treated.
Catheterization period: 149-598 days, average 374 days,
number of sepsis: 3 or 27.3 %.
Blood culture: Serratia marcescens, Pseudomonas sp., S. aureus.

The most frequent microorganisms responsible for catheter infections and proven catheter-related sepsis in our patients are seen in Table 1.

Table 1. Microorganisms cultured from catheter tip/blood.

	HD catheter		
	Femoral	Subclavian	Francis
S. Aureus	IIIIIII	IIIIIIIII	I
S. Epidermis	III	IIIIIII	
Proteus sp.		II	
Acitenobacter sp.		I	
Nef Gram neg.*		II	
E. coli	II		
Enterobacter sp.	I		
Pseudomonas sp.	I		I
Serr. marcescens			I

* non fermentive Gram negative bacteria

Sepsis Treatment

We removed the catheter or changed the site of insertion and we used antibiotics. Three patients of 35 died. Sepsis may have contributed but wasn't the main cause of death. One patient had systemic vasculitis and pneumonia, two patients had meta Ca mammae and Ca recti and ESRD.

S. aureus und S. epidermidis were the most common microbial isolates found on 38 catheter sepsis episodes in our patients and those described by other authors [2, 3].

Although septic, our patients had a low mortality, an observation previously noted by other investigators too [4]. No morbis events (e.g. bacterial endocarditis, metastatic infections) and no deaths could be attributed to the catheter-related sepsis.

In our study comparing infection rates in subclavian catheter, tunneled or not tunneled, we found significant differences in catheter sepsis incidence: 1.9 % in tunneled versus 5.9 % in non tunneled subclavian catheters. This in contrast to results, reported by Dahlberg et al. [5].

Conclusions

Femoral dialysis catheters are associated with a low incidence of sepsis. The major cause appears to be a rigorous local site care in an immobile patient done by experienced dialysis medical staff.

Infectious complications from subclavian catheters exceed those with femoral catheters, especially non tunneled. Therefore we can recommend subcutaneous tunneling of catheters.

The incidence of sepsis with Francis catheters is much higher, but the main reason is a long period of catheterization. Treatment of sepsis was successful.

References

[1] HAKIN, R. M., J. M. LAZARUS: Medical aspects of hemodialysis, pp. 1791-1845. In: BRENNER, B. M., F. C. RECTOR (eds.): The kidney. W. B. Saunders: Philadelphia 1986.

[2] CHEESBROUGH, J. S., R. G. FINCH, R. P. BURDEN: A Prospective Study of the Mechanisms of Infection Associated with Hemodialysis Catheters. *J. Infect. Dis.* 154: no. 4 (1986).

[3] MOYER, M. A., L. D. EDWARDS, L. FARLEY: Comparative Culture Methods on 101 Intravenous Catheters. *Arch. Intern. Med.* 143: Jan. (1983).

[4] KOZENY, G. A., F. R. VENEZIO, V. K. BANSAL, L. L. VERTUNO, J. E. HANO: Incidence of Subclavian Dialysis Catheter – Related Infections. *Arch. Intern. Med.* 144: Sept. (1984).

[5] DAHLBERG, P. J., W. R. YULUC, K. L. NEWCOMER: Subclavian Hemodialysis Catheter Infections. *Am. J. Kidney Dis.* 7: no. 5 (1986).

Catheter Technology: Biocompatibility

A Comparison of Different Preparatory Methods of Blood Cells for Investigation with the Scanning Electron Microscope

D. BEHREND, D. FALKENHAGEN, G. S. BROWN, G. DREWS,
H.-P. PUTZKE, H. KLINKMANN

Abstract

Based on considerations and a critical review of preparation methods for investigations with the scanning electron microscope found in the literature, a standard method for sample preparation was developed which allowed an adequate cell representation without damaging polymer biomaterial coatings. It could be demonstrated that drying in air of fixed blood cells subsequent to dehydration with ethanol and ether was no more traumatic for the cells than critical point drying. Furthermore drying in air has the advantage that it requires less time and technical equipment than for instance critical point drying and contamination of the samples with amyl acetate or waste products from the CO_2 bomb can be avoided.

Introduction

The surface morphology of a biomaterial following contact with blood is of critical importance for the assessment of the in vitro and in vivo biocompatibility of the material of interest. Morphological investigations can be performed using light optical methods and scanning electron microscopy. Light optical methods such as reflection microscopy or phase contrast microscopy in transmission mode are limited in their resolution of objects and impose the precondition that the substrate is permeable to light.
The scanning electron microscopy (SEM) provides the method of choice for tackling the above mentioned problems. Using this method it is possible to obtain a pseudoplastic image of cellular blood elements on the surface of a biomaterial with a wide magnification range infinitely adjustable. Events preceeding the adhesion and spreading of platelets as well as alterations in the cell morphology, e.g. of white blood cells, can be readily identified with the aid of the SEM [1-3].
A preparatory method which is gentle and reproducible is a critical requirement for scanning electron micrographs of cells adhering to a biomaterial [16].
Several suggestions concerning the preparation of blood cells for SEM investigations are to be found in the scientific literature, however, such descriptions are generally

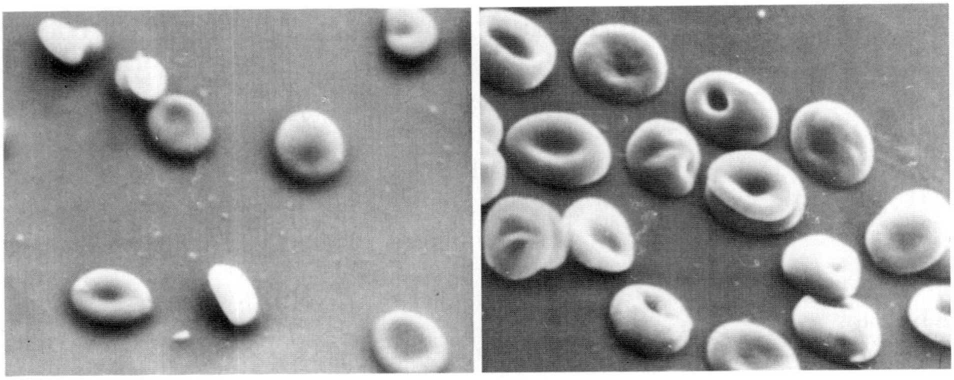

Fig. 1-2. Human erythrocytes prepared according to Method 1-2.

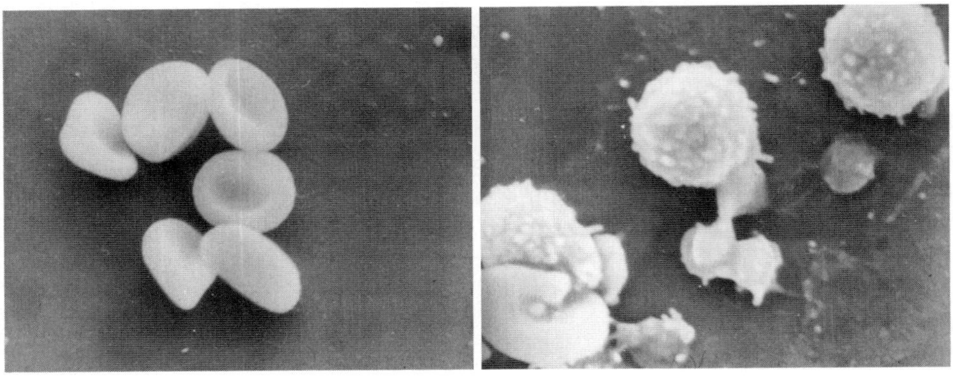

Fig. 3-4. Human erythrocytes and leukocytes prepared according to Method 3.

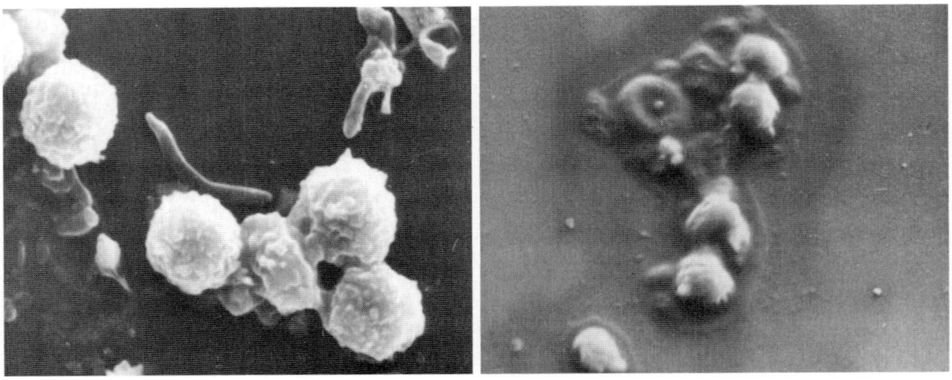

Fig. 5-6. Human erythrocytes, leukocytes and thrombocytes prepared according to Method 4, artifacts following critical point drying.

short and incomplete [4-6]. The matter is further complicated by the observed qualitative differences in results obtained from electron micrographs of samples prepared using the same method [17-19].

The aim of this study was to investigate the applicability of selected, recognized preparation methods using freshly collected human whole blood and to develop a standard method tailored to meet the requirements set by the available technical possibilities. These standard methods were essential for further, more intensive investigations which required incontestable scanning electron micrographs of cellular blood components. The method was to be suitable for both human blood samples and blood from the animal species generally used in our biomaterial research program namely rat and dog. In this way both blood samples following contact with an artificial surface and blood samples not brought into contact with an artificial surface could be examined and any differences in morphology identified.

Materials and Methods

Prior to a scanning electron microscope investigation blood cells and tissues must undergo four steps:

1. cell separation
2. fixation
3. dehydration/drying
4. sputtering

The initial processing step is only necessary for investigations of blood cells from whole blood in the absence of biomaterial contact or cells obtained from a cell culture. It is naturally not necessary in the case of biomaterial samples following blood contact.

Whole blood anticoagulated with EDTA, heparin, or sodium citrate (preferentially the latter) is centrifuged for 10 min at 60 g. Details for the centrifugation procedure vary in the literature between 50 and 650 g and 6-10 min [7-9]. A lower/shorter centrifugation condition is less traumatic for the cells, however, higher centrifugation conditions result in improved separation.

The 2nd step is necessary to avoid any permanent changes to the cell volume and surface. Through fixation it is hoped that the macromolecular cellular scaffolding is stabilized through the immersion or perfusion into the sample of various agents [7, 10]. The most commonly used agents are:

- glutaraldehyde
- osmium tetraoxide
- formaldehyde
- acrolein
- ethanol

- uranyl acetate
- quick silver dichloride (sublimate)

Glutaraldehyde fixation results in a good preservation of structure due to bridging incorporating several C atoms between the amino groups of lysine and through reactions with aromatic amino acids leading to intra- and intermolecular bonds between proteins and thus a very fine protein denaturation [7, 10, 16]. Glutaraldehyde is, however, taken up very slowly by the cells. Osmium tetraoxide is the only fixation agent which does not result in shrinkage at the low concentrations used [7]. It results in rapid cell fixation due to a fast infiltration of the cell, C=C bonding to unsaturated fatty acids resulting in bridge formation which in turn gives rise to a lipid network. The storage of osmium furthermore leads to an increased contrast and a reduction in charge artifacts. Rinsing the sample is an important step subsequent to any chemical fixation. Phosphate buffered saline [11] or, less often, aqua bidest, is generally used.

The dehydration step must be carried out before drying to prevent alterations to the surface and volume of the cell subsequent to the chemical fixation. The cell water is replaced by a fluid with a significantly lower surface energy. Ethanol and acetone are such fluids. Ethanol is most frequently selected for use due not only to its low surface energy but also because of its ability to mix with water. It can be considered furthermore to some extent a postfixation agent. It dissolves, however, fats and waxes out of the cell membrane thus in order to preserve fine surface structures, a prior treatment with osmium tetraoxide is recommended.

Ethanol also results in cell shrinkage and for this reason the dehydration time should be kept as short as possible. The increasing ethanol concentrations and submersion times of the sample in ethanol which are given in the literature vary greatly. The most frequent recommendation is 5-10 min immersion in 20, 50, 95 and 100 % ethanol solution [20-23]. For minimal shrinkage immersion for 10 min in 15, 30, 40, 60, 70, 80, 90, 95 and 100 % ethanol solution is recommended. The increased time required for this must be balanced out with the improved quality of the sample. The sample may be dried according to three procedures:

- air,
- critical point drying (CPD),
- freeze drying.

Of these methods, drying in air and CPD have received the most international acclaim [11-13]. A procedure using a mixture of ethanol and ether has been reported to cause minimal trauma to the cells [7]. CPD can be performed with CO_2, freon or dinitrogen oxide, whereby freon 13 is the most frequently used method [7, 19]. In comparison to samples prepared by alternative drying methods, samples prepared by freeze drying are reported to shrink by only 7-9 % [14]. A disadvantage of this method is the time required to prepare samples and the freeze dried sample must be kept in a vacuum and immediately sputtered due to their high hydroscopicity [7].

Table 1. Assessment scheme for the preparation methods.

Method	Fixation	Rinsing	Post-Fixation	Rinsing	Dehydration	Drying
1	2.5 % GA 4.0 % GA	Water	– –	– –	Ethanol/ Water	AC/CPD
2	2.5 % GA 4.0 % GA	PBS	0.5 % OsO_4	Water	–	Air
3	2.5 % GA 4.0 % GA	PBS	0.5 % OsO_4	Water	Ethanol/ Ether	Air
4	2.5 % GA 4.0 % GA	PBS	0.5 % OsO_4	Water	Ethanol/ Water	AC / CPD
5	2.5 % GA 4.0 % GA	PBS	0.5 % OsO_4 Water saturated sublimate	Water	Ethanol/ Ether	Air
6	2.5 % GA 4.0 % GA	PBS	0.5 % OsO_4 Water saturated sublimate	Water	Ethanol/ Water	AC / CPD
7	Freon	–	–	–	–	GFT
8	DMSO	–	–	–	–	GFT

GA : Glutaraldehyde; AC : Amylacetate; OsO_4 : Osmium tetraoxide;
CPD : Critical point drying; PBS : Phosphate buffer saline;
GFT : Freeze drying; Freon : Cooling solution;
DMSO : Dimethyl sulfoxide as frost protection medium

Prior to sputtering the following treatment has proved to be advantageous. The fixed and dried sample should initially be mounted on a glass carrier which has previously been treated with gold and coated with 0.001 % poly-L-lysine solution which is then placed in the metal sample carrier and the joining edges sealed with silver. The subsequent sputtering is performed with carbon and gold until a coating is achieved with a thickness of 80-100 nm in a pre-vacuum of 0.1 torr.
The aim of our investigations was to compare as far as possible the methods given in the literature due to short and incomplete description, with one another and with our newly developed methods in an attempt to obtain an optimal standard sample preparation technique.
The various steps which were performed to develop a standard method are shown in Table 1. Fresh human blood was prepared according to these methods and blood cells from our most frequently used animal models (rat-Wistar, ROZT, Beagle) were prepared according to the developed standard preparation method.

Results

It is intended to critically discuss and compare all the methods listed in Table 1. It is acknowledged [7] that the red blood cells are the most sensitive of all blood cells to the preparation method. The red blood cells prepared according to Method 1 are round. Approximately 20 % are biconcaval disks and the remainder have heavily

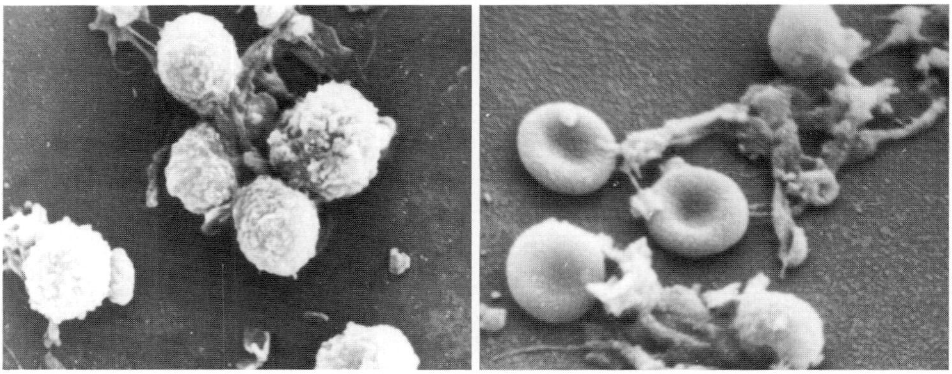

Fig. 7-8. Human erythrocytes, leukocytes and thrombocytes prepared according to Method 5-6.

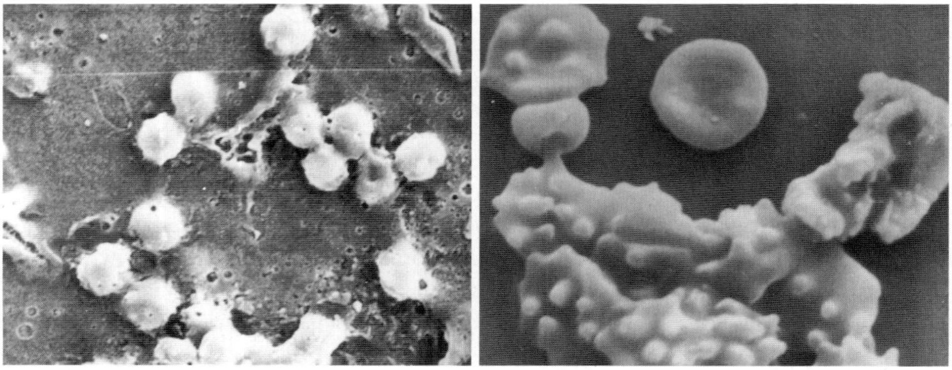

Fig. 9-10. Human erythrocytes and leukocytes prepared according to Method 7-8.

thickened circumferences and round forms (Fig. 1) which may be explained by the absence of a postfixation step with osmium tetraoxide. It may be concluded that the lipid network plays an important role in preserving the form of erythrocytes. Method 2 is similarly not completely satisfactory. Here the evaporated tissue fluid, resulting from the high surface energy, causes a surface change in the form of small undulating outgrowths on normal erythrocytes from healthy donors. Only approximately 40 % of erythrocytes are to be observed in their normal form using this preparation technique (Fig. 2). Surprisingly good results were obtained with Method 3 (Fig. 3, 4).

Method 4 is the method most frequently described in the literature and employing this method one obtains results qualitatively similar to those obtained with Method 3 (Fig. 5, 6). Surface differentiations between white blood cells and platelets can be clearly depicted. It should, however, be noted that artifacts often arise when this method is applied. These take the form of oily films and clear contamination of the cells and may be assigned to the amyl acetate used. With respect to a fine depiction of blood cell surface structures, Method 5 is superior to both Methods 3 and 4. Using this method filopodien-like outgrowths as well as diverse spreading forms of platelets are readily distinguishable (Fig. 7). The reason for this lies in the use of sublimate for postfixation enabling additional intra- and intermolecular bonds to form due to the formation of stable chelatocomplexes of quick silver between the carboxyl amino groups or imidazole rests as ligands. This results in a stable binding of proteins, lipoproteins and lipids near to the surface so that upon exposure to ethanol hardly any membrane lipids and lipoproteins can be removed. As expected, results similar to those obtained with Method 5 were obtained with Method 6 (Fig. 8). The granulation in the background observed with Methods 5 and 6 is due to precoating with the substrate carrier poly-L-lysine. The results obtained with Method 7 were unsatisfactory but this can be explained by the variations in the method description given in the literature. The results obtained with Method 8 must be similarly assessed. The majority of erythrocytes are to be found in the crenated cell form (Fig. 10) due to the effect of DMSO.

Discussion

The scanning electron micrographs shown in Figures 1, 2 and 10 indicate that Methods 1, 2 and 8 are not suitable for the preparation of blood cells. If Method 1 is selected then postfixation with OsO_4 must be performed otherwise charge artifacts arise. Method 2 which involves the simple drying in air of non-dehydrated cells demonstrated that the surface and volume changes arising from evaporation can not be compensated by a postfixation step with OsO_4. Freezing cells with dimethyl sulfoxide leads to alterations in permeability properties of the cells the results of which can be serious due to the effect of DMSO as a cell poison.

It could be demonstrated that Methods 3, 4, 5, and 6 are suitable preparatory methods for cells for scanning electron microscope investigations. Method 5 is favored for future investigations and furthermore its use recommended despite the fact that Method 4 is almost exclusively the method of choice in the international literature. Drying in air following dehydration with ethanol and ether exposes the fixed blood cells to equally as little trauma as critical point drying and is technically simpler. If critical point drying is chosen then the possibility arises that the samples will be contaminated with amylacetate or with waste products from the CO_2 bomb. Comparatively good results could most certainly be obtained with Method 7 if a suitable lyophiliser capable of high quality freeze drying is available. The time and instrumentation required for this method is, however, much greater than that for Method 5. Method 5 is recommended as standard preparation method which

Table 2. Methods of preparation of cellular blood components.

Methods	Picture Quality	Accuracy	Artifact Frequency	Technical Complexity	Time necessary	Usefulness
1	(+)	+	+++	++	+++	–
2	+	+	+++	+	+	–
3	++	++	(+)	+	+	+
4	++	++	++	++	++	+
5	+++	+++	(+)	+	+	+++
6	+++	++	++	++	++	++
7	(++)*	(++)*	(+++)	+++	+++	(+)*
8	+	+	+++	+++	+++	–

helps achieve high quality representation of blood cells or biomaterial test-bodies subsequent to biomaterial contact.

A qualitative assessment scheme for each of the methods investigated is given in Table 2.

References

[1] Schakenraad, J. M., J. Arends, H. J. Buseler, P. B. Von Wachern, C. R. H. Wildevuur: Kinetics of cell spreading on protein precoated substrate – a study of interfacial aspects. *Biomaterials* 10: 43-50 (1989).

[2] Lowenberg, B. F., R. M. Pilliar, J. E. Ausin, J. Sodek, A. H. Melder: Cell attachment of human gingival fibroblasts in vitro toporous-surfaced titanium alloy discs coated with collagen and platelet-drived growth factor. *Biomaterials* 9: 302-309 (1988).

[3] Goodman, S. L., T. G. Grasel, S. L. Cooper, R. M. Albrecht: Platelet shape change and cytoskeletal reorganization on polyurethaneureas. *J. Biomed. Mat. Res.* 23: 105-123 (1989).

[4] McCoy, T. G., H. D. Wobers, S. L. Cooper: Series shunt evaluation of polyurethane vascular growth materials in chronically AV-shunted canines. *J. Biomed. Mat. Res.* 24: 107-129 (1990).

[5] Seifert, L. M., R. T. Greer: Evaluation of in vivo adsorption of blood elements onto hydrogel – coated silicone rubber by SEM and fourier transform infrared spectroscopy. *J. Biomed. Mat. Res.* 19: 1043-1071 (1985).

[6] Baier, R. R., V. A. DePalma, D. w. goupil, E. Cohen: Human platelet spreading on substrata of Known surface chemistry. *J. Biomed. Mat. Res.* 19: 1157-1167 (1985).

[7] Rosenbauer, K. A., B. H. Kegel (eds.): Rasterelektonenmikroskopische Techniken in der Medizin und Biologie. Thieme: Stuttgart 1978.

[8] Whithouse, W. H.: Indium – 111 – oxine labeled platelet imaging of endothelial seeded dacron thoraco – abdominal vascular prosthesis in a canine model. *Trans. Am. Soc. Artif. Int. Organs* 29: 183-185 (1983).

[9] Bernstein, E. F., V. M. Marzec, T. E. Johnston: Structural correlations of platelet funktional damage by physical forces. *Trans. Am. Soc. Artif. Int. Organs* 23: 617-625 (1977).

[10] Ruzicka, F.: Elektronenmikroskopische Hämatologie. Springer: Wien 1976.

[11] Mason, R. G., B. A. Shinode: Reaction of blood with artificial surfaces of hemodialyzes studies of human blood with platelet defects or coagulation factor deficiencies. *Biomaterials* 6: 305-329 (1978).

[12] ALBRECHT, R. M., S. L. GOODMAN, S. R. SIMMONS: Distribution and movement of membrane-associated platelet glycoproteins: use of colloidal gold with correlative videoenhanced light microscopy, low-voltage high-resolution scanning electron microscopy, and high-voltage transmissionelectron microscopy. *The American Journal of Anatomy* 185: 149-164 (1989).

[13] GOODMAN, S. L., R. M. ALBRECHT: Correlative light and electron microscopy of platelet adhesion and fibrinogen receptor expression using colloidal-gold labeling. *Scan. Microsc.* 1: 727-734 (1987).

[14] DAGALAKIS, N., J. FLINK, P. STASIKELIS, J. F. BURKE: Design of an artificial skin. Part III. Control of pore structure. *J. Biomed. Mat. Res.* 14: 511-528 (1980).

[15] DREWS, G.: Methode zur Entwicklung einer Präparation von Blutzellen für die rasterelektronenmikroskopische Darstellung. Diplomarbeit Universität Rostock, Fakultät für Medizin, 1989.

[16] MCNAMARA, A., D. F. WILLIAMS: Scanning electron microscopy of the metal-tissue interface. *Biomaterials* 3: 160-164 (1982).

[17] FUJITA, T. K., J. TANAKA, J. TOKUNAGA (eds.): SEM-atlas of cells and tissues. Igaku-Shoin: Tokyo 1981.

[18] MARCHANT, R. E., J. M. ANDERSON, K. PHUA, A. HILTNER: In vivo biocompatibility studies, 2. Biomer. Preliminary cell adhesion and surface characterization studies. *J. Biomed. Mat. Res.* 16: 471-500 (1982).

[19] VALE, B. H., R. T. GREER: Ex vivo shunt testing of hydrogen – silicone rubber composite materials. *J. Biomed. Mat. Res.* 16: 471-500 (1982).

[20] EBERHARD, R. C., M. E. LYNCH, F. M. BILGE, M. A. ARTS: Effects of fluid shear and temperature on protein adsorption on teflon surfaces. *Trans. Am. Soc. Artif. Int. Organs* 26: 185-187 (1980).

[21] LEE, R. S., S. W. KIM: Adsorbed glycoproteins in platelet adhesion onto polymer surfaces: Significance to terminal galactose units. *Trans. Am. Soc. Artif. Int. Organs* 26: 511-528 (1980).

[22] MASON, R. G., B. A. SHINODE: Reaction of blood with artificial surfaces of hemodialyzers studies of human blood with platelet defects or coagulation factor deficiencies. *Biomaterials* 6: 305-329 (1978).

[23] DAHLKE, H., N. DOCIN, K. THURAU: Thrombogenicity of different suture materials by scanningelectron microscopy. *J. Biomed. Mat. Res.* 14: 251-268 (1980).

Scanning Electron Microscopy of Large Bore Catheters

P. MESTRES, R. BAMBAUER, U. WEBER

Abstract

Catheter embolism, thrombosis, thromboembolism and infection are serious complications following the use of intravascular catheters in humans. In such pathological processes the material used, the surface characteristics and the design of the catheters play an important role. In the present study the scanning electron microscope was used to examine the surface of the catheters before and after implantation in patients. The following types of materials were investigated: Teflon, polypropylene, polyurethane and carbon coated polyurethane. Short catheter segments were opened longitudinally, fixed, dehydrated and critical point dried. After coating with gold, both inner and outer surfaces were examined in a scanning electron microscope.

Considerable differences in the surface structure between implanted and non-implanted catheters were observed. Teflon catheters show the inner surface with numerous longitudinal microgrooves and at the outer surfaces small pits and hollows. In the polypropylene catheters both surfaces appear unevenly configured with numerous pits randomly distributed. In contrast, the polyurethane catheters present very smooth surfaces and sharp borders at the lateral holes.

Differences in the interaction with blood were observed depending on the type of implanted catheter. Signs of thrombogenic reaction were observed earlier on the polyurethane and polypropylene than on the Teflon or carbon coated catheters.

Table 1. Investigated catheters.

Catheter	Material	Number of samples
Cath-line	Polyurethane	12
Cath-line	Carbon-coated Polyurethane	11
Vascath	Teflon (radio-opaque)	7
Uni-cath	Polypropylene	10

These observations are of interest in two concerns: one is the control of materials used for manufacturing catheters and second is the catheter surface interactions with the blood. Both aspects are important in order to determine the suitability of catheters for clinical purposes.

Introduction

The use of intravascular catheters in humans is frequently the origin of serious clinical complications as for example, infections, catheter embolism, thrombosis and thromboembolism [1]. Whereas embolic complications seem to be dependent of implantation performance, thrombosis and thromboembolism are related with some catheter attributes like the material used, surface structure and catheter design [2-5]. In the same order of things the adhesion properties of the catheter surfaces may likewise play a role in the adhesion of bacteria and microbial colonization [6]. For these reasons the selection of material and procedure for manufacturing catheters is an important matter.

Table 2. Scanning Electron Microscopy (schedule).

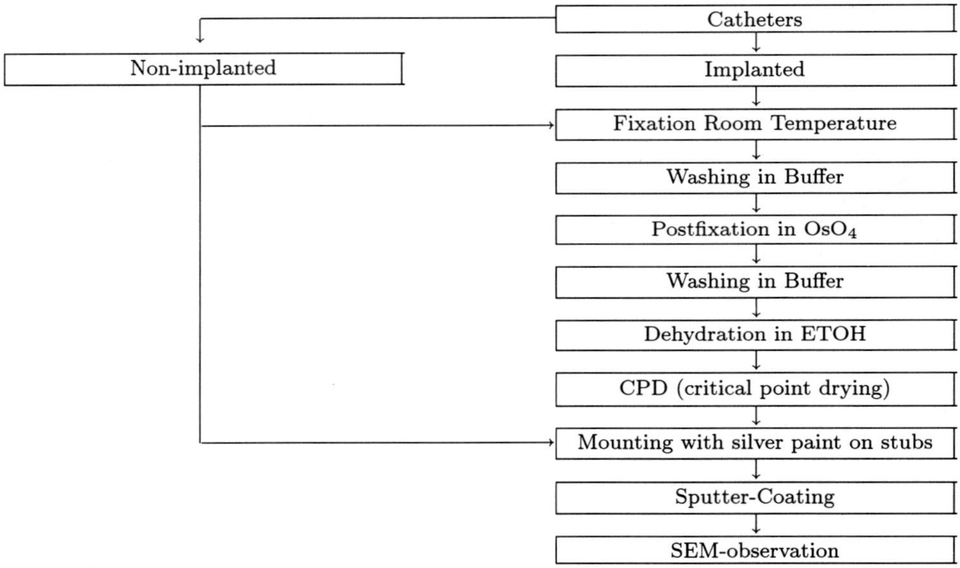

A number of methods are available for examination of surfaces of materials proposed for contact with flowing blood. These methods concern the analysis of surface parameters (surface textures, charge and chemistry) and the study of thrombogenic reactions as well [7]. One of the techniques that cover many aspects of this area is the scanning electron microscopy (SEM). First of all, the SEM allows the study of catheter surfaces showing the degree of roughness, i.e., the existence of cracks, fissures and valleys that are more or less filled with air or liquids in microscopical quantities, which may influence the interactions between blood and the catheter wall [7]. Secondly, the behavior of the blood on the catheter surfaces is surely an important determinant for their suitability [8]. The thrombogenic character of a surface may be documented by SEM showing for instance the attachment and morphology of blood cell aggregates or the formation of fibrin cables and thrombi.

Considering this background, we have used the SEM to describe the structure of four types of catheters currently used in our hospital and at the same time to estimate the thrombogenicity or thromboresistance of their surfaces implanted in patients.

Material and Methods

The structure of the surfaces was investigated in non-implanted sterile catheters (Table 1). These specimens were examined directly i.e. without any special treatment, but some others were treated for control purposes according with the same schedule of the implanted ones.

The implanted catheters used by patients were prepared for SEM following a schedule proposed by [1] but slightly modified for our purposes (Table 2). Segments of 0.5 cm length divided into longitudinal halves were fixed by immersion in a buffered solution containing 3 % glutaraldehyde and 1 % formaldehyde [9]. For examination in the scanning electron microscope the specimens were mounted exposing one half the inner and the other half the outer surface. At least two lateral holes were included within the selected segments. The specimens were coated with gold (5-10 nm thick) in a Balzers sputter apparatus and examined in a CamScan S2 scanning electron microscope at 10 kV.

Results

Scanning electron microscopy of non-implanted catheters.

Considerable differences in the surface structure of the four catheter types were observed. The Teflon catheter has in the entire length an inner surface with small furrows or microgrooves and thin ridges along the longitudinal axis (Fig. 1). The lateral holes were in general not cleanly punched and display a more or less irregular configuration (Fig. 2). In the outer surfaces of this catheter type small pits, microcavities and irregular defects were found. The polypropylene catheter has an irregular surface morphology with numerous pits and an unevenly configurated inner and outer faces (Figs. 3-4). Like the Teflon catheter, the polypropylene catheter has lateral holes with unclean punched borders. The polyurethane catheters have very smooth faces with practically no pits. The edges of the lateral holes show clean cuted borders. The polyurethane catheters coated with carbon display basically the same surface characteristics as the uncoated and seem to be more sensitive against dehydrating agents (not shown).

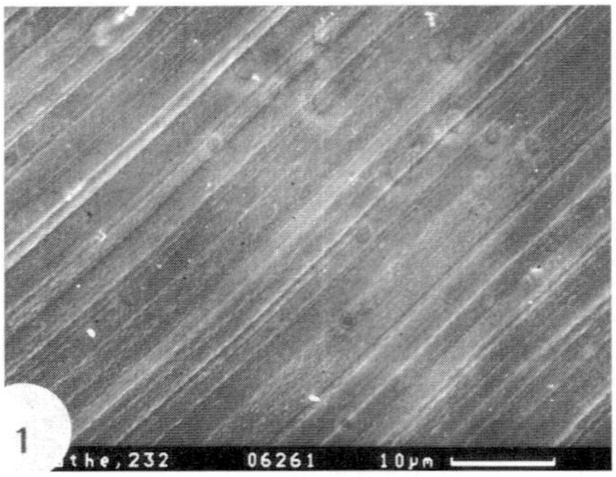

Fig. 1. Inner face of a Teflon catheter. Note the longitudinal microgrooves.

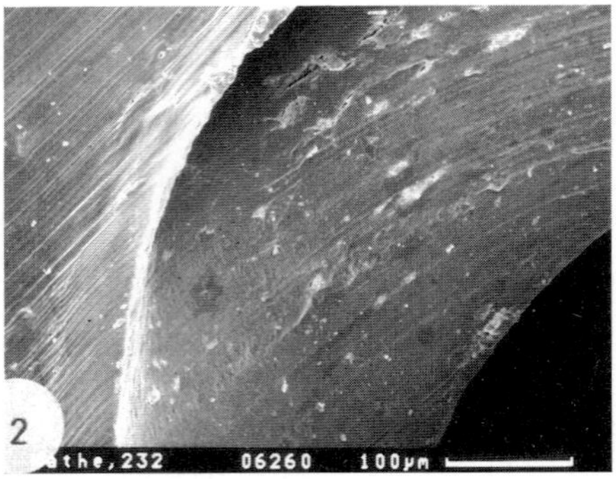

Fig. 2. Detail of a lateral hole of a Teflon catheter. Note the configuration of borders.

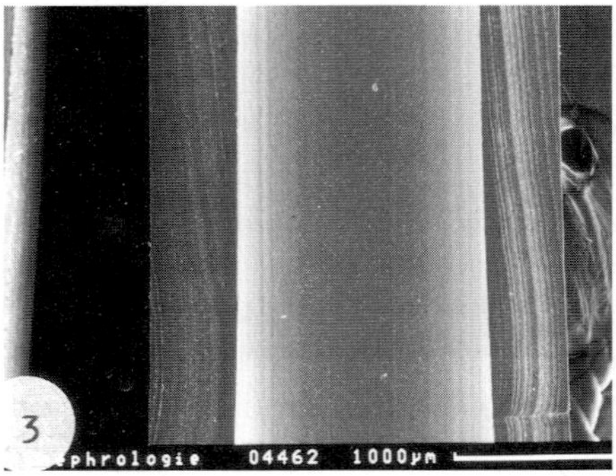

Fig. 3. Catheter opened longitudinally (polypropylene).

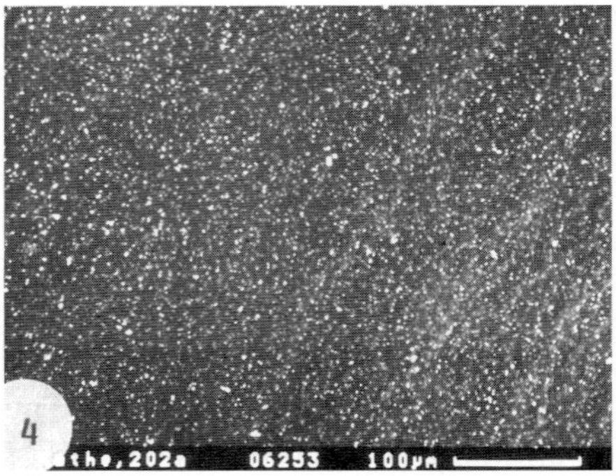

Fig. 4. Detail of Fig. 3. Note the numerous pits of the surface.

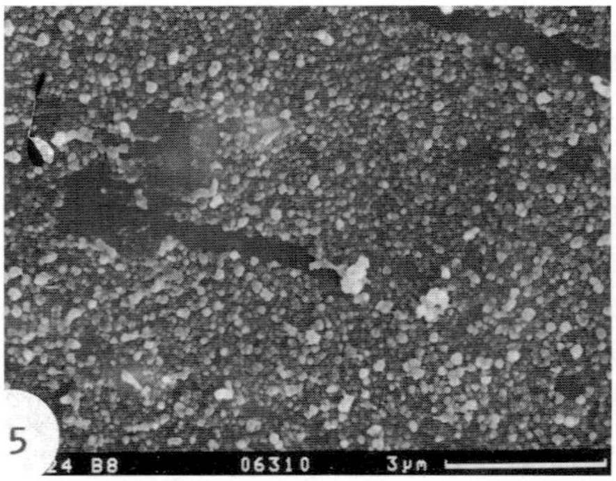

Fig. 5. Surface of a catheter (PU=polyurethane) coated by small globules and particles of proteinaceous material. This is a case of thick coating.

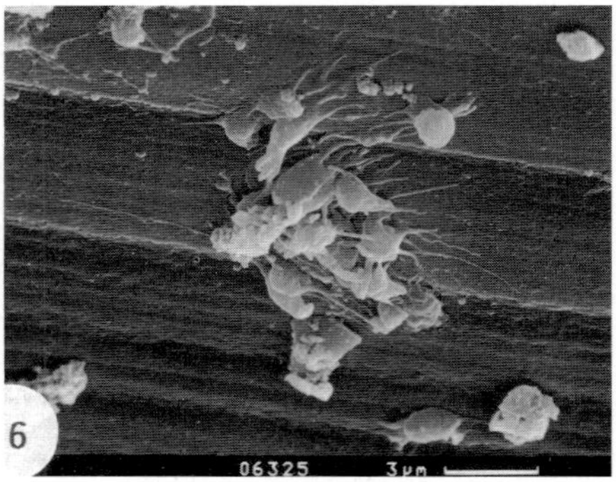

Fig. 6. Platelets attached to the catheter surface (PU). Note the existence of filopodia and other cell extensions typical for platelets during the phase of spreading out.

Scanning electron microscopy of implanted catheters.

A careful inspection with the SEM of catheters implanted for 24 hours, reveals that their surfaces are covered by a thin layer of a protein-like material (Fig. 5). Large areas of the catheter surfaces show no longer the textural features above described. Instead one found numerous granules and very small particles attached to the inner surfaces. On the Teflon and carbon coated polyurethane catheters the proteinaceous coat seems to be thinner than in the polypropylene and uncoated polyurethane catheters. The outer surfaces show a coating as well, but more heterogeneous probably because the diversity of tissues in contact.

Table 3. Chronology of the thrombogenic events.

Catheter	conditioning*	cell attachment	fibrin cables	clotting
Teflon	1	4-7	10	14-15
Polypropylene	1	2-4	2-4	4-6
Polyurethane	1	1	5	7-10
Polyurethane carbon-coated	1	3-5	5-7	10

*: Days after implantation.

After this early period, one can find depending of catheter type, signs of thrombogenesis, for instance, the attachment of cells, the formation of a meshwork of fibrin cables and trapped erythrocytes. The fibrin clots are in the initial stages laminar in shape, and depending of time, they may reach a considerable thickness. In such situations obstructions of the lateral holes are frequent. The more characteristic events of thrombogenic reaction observed in our material are documented in the case of the polyurethane catheter (Figs. 6-10). The platelets become adherent and in some cases they can develope thin and long filopodia (Fig. 6.) Also leukocytes and specially monocytes appear attached and often arranged like a monolayer (Fig. 7). At higher magnification the monocytes show typical cell borders with flattened or/and finger-like extensions (Fig. 8). Finally it is possible to see in some catheter preparations, depending how long were implanted, several stages of the formation of thrombi (Figs. 9-10).

A comparison of the chronological evolution of the thrombogenesis allows to detect some differences between catheters used in this investigation (Table 3). Cell attachment and clotting was detected earlier in the polypropylene catheters than in the other types. It is remarkable that in the Teflon and carbon coated polyurethane catheters the thrombogenic reaction seems to progress more slowly than in the other types. These observations suggest that Teflon has a better thromboresistence. Also the carbon coating of the polyurethane catheters seem to modify favorably the thromboresistence of this material.

Concerning the microbial contamination, only in three cases bacterial colonies were observed (not shown), a really low rate.

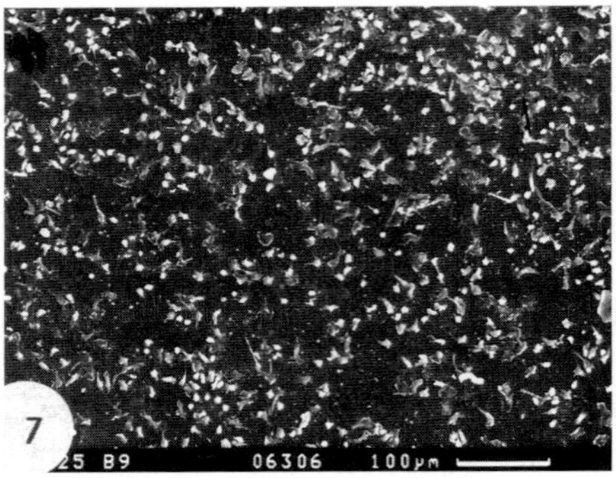

Fig. 7. Adhesion of leukocytes and monocytes during the early period of implantation (polyurethane). In this area practically no other cells appear attached to the surface.

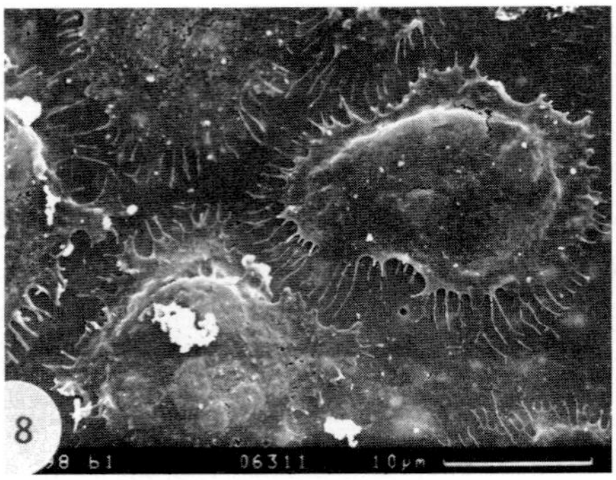

Fig. 8. Monocytes at higher magnification (polyurethane). Note the very characteristic shape of the cell borders.

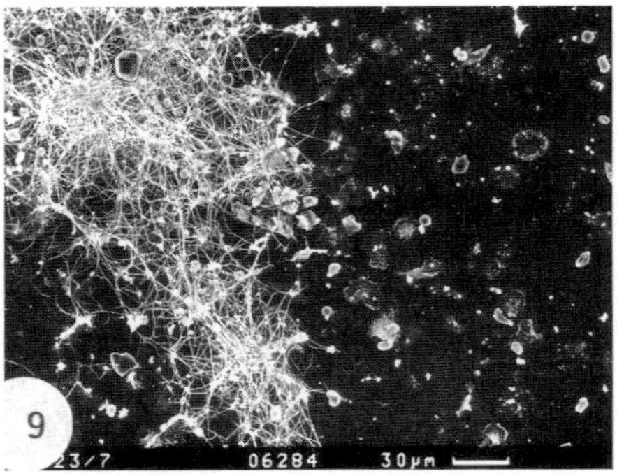

Fig. 9. During the thromobogenesis one see fibrin cables intermingled with monocytes and leukocytes (polyurethane).

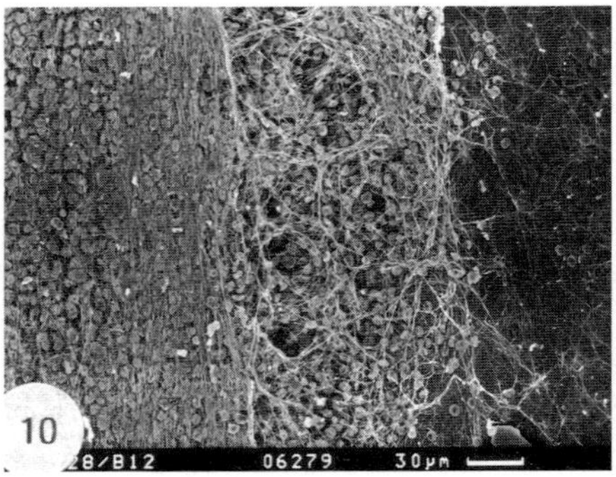

Fig. 10. Thrombus with a luminal thin layer of fibrin (polyurethane).

Discussion

The four types of catheters investigated show remarkable differences in their surface structures. In agreement with previous studies of other groups the polyurethane catheters are rather smooth [1, 4, 10]. However, after carbon coating the roughness of their surfaces is increased, probably because the coating conditions. In contrast, the polypropylene catheters have surfaces with a high degree of roughness [10]. The Teflon catheters although they don't have a flattened surface also can not be considered as rough for two reasons: first, because the orderly arrangement of the microgrooves and second, because the smoothness of the microgrooves. Therefore this type of catheter should be classified as less rough than others.
Frequently, in the literature, one mentione alterations of catheter surface due it to the action of chemical agents used in the preparation for SEM (for literature see [1]).

Table 4. Thrombogenic Reaction on Catheters (sequence of events observed with the SEM).

I.	surface conditioning
II.	cell attachment (platelet attachment)
III.	attachment of leukocytes
IV.	thrombosis: – early – later stages (with occlusion of lateral holes and formation of tunneled thrombi)

Table 5. Molecular aspects of the thrombogenic reaction.

surface conditioning:	plasma proteins (cell adhesion proteins)
platelets attachment:	fibrinogen vitronectine Willebrand factor fibronectine
leukocytes attachment:	complement (C3) activation denaturation of conditioning film
thrombosis	

Most of the artifacts attributable to the dehydration were observed in our material only after very long periods of treatment with alcohols. This type of alterations may be avoided using the dehydrating agent (ethanol, methanol...) at temperatures between 0°-4° C. In this context it is interesting to mention that catheters coated with proteins, for instance with serum, and then fixed with aldehydes and osmium tetraoxide, are much more stable against the dehydrating agents [8].

The behavior of the blood elements indicates that they react with a surface depending of its grade of roughness [7, 11]. However, the chemical characteristics of the surfaces may play a additional role at the onset and during the thrombogenic reaction (Table 4 and 5). In general, the plasma proteins should react with the catheter constituing a thin protein film, a process called surface conditioning [7]. The behavior of the blood cells, particularly during the initial phase of the thrombogenic reaction, could be close related with the structure and composition of the this conditioning film. Thus the adhesion of platelets could be related with the absorption of fibrinogen into this film [12-16]. On the other hand, the attachment of leukocytes and monocytes could be expression of the complement activation, in which the fragment C3 is able to increase the cell adhesion and/or be related with the presence of fibronectin in the conditioning film [16]. A denaturation of the proteins of the conditioning film can also increase the cell adhesion. This sequence of events were registered in all four types of catheters, but differences were observed in the timing. Although we cannot confirm statistically the significance of these

differences, it is important to note again that the onset of thrombogenic reaction appear delayed in some of these catheters.
In conclusion, the SEM provides valuable information about conditioning of catheter surfaces and about their thrombogenic properties. The behavior of the blood cells particularly during the early phases of the blood-catheter interactions reveals that they are conditions and that in this phenomenon diverse cell adhesion proteins of the blood are involved.

References

[1] Rosenbauer, K. A.: Light microscopic and scanning microscopic findings on intravenous polyurethane catheters. In: Johari, O. (ed.): Scanning Electron Microscopy / 1982/II (Pages 765-772), SEM Inc. MFA O'Hare (Chicago, III.).

[2] Mason, R. G., D. E. Scarborough, S. R. Saba, K. M. Brinkhous, L. D. Ikenberry, J. J. Kearney, H. G. Clark: Thrombogenicity of some biomedical materials: Platelet-interface Reactions. *J. Biomed. Mater. Res.* 3: 615-644 (1969).

[3] Burri, C., H. Henkemeyer, H. H. Passler: Katheterembolien. *Schweiz. Med. Wschr.* 101: 1537-1544 (1971).

[4] Rosenbauer, K. A., J. A. Herzer, B. Jansen: Scanning electron microscopic studies of different types of intravenous catheters before and after usage. *Acta Anat.* 111: 129-130 (1981).

[5] Bambauer, R., G. A. Jutzler: Transcutaneous insertion of the Shaldon catheter through the internal jugular vein as access for acute hemodialysis. *Dial. Transplant.* 11: 766-773 (1982).

[6] Peters, G.: Plastikinfektionen durch Staphylokokken. *Dt. Ärztebl.* 86: 234-239 (1988).

[7] Baier, R. E.: Selected methods of investigation for Blood-Contact surfaces. *Ann. N. Y. Acad. Sci.* 516: 68-77 (1987).

[8] Hoffman, A. S.: Modification of material surfaces to affect how they interact with blood. *Ann. N.Y. Acad. Sci.* 516: 96-101 (1987).

[9] Mestres, P., K. Rascher, A. Garfia: Bedeutung und Perspektiven des REM in Neuroanatomie und experimentelle Neuropathologie. *Beiträge zur Elektronenmikroskopischen Direktabbildung von Oberflächen (BEDO)* 13: 165-276 (1980).

[10] Bambauer, R., P. Mestres, U. Weber: Raster electron microscopic (REM) investigations in large bore catheters for extracorporeal detoxification. Int. Symp. on Optimization of Bloodpurification. Rostock-Warnemünde, Sept. 1987. *Int. Soc. Artif. Organs.*

[11] Merril, E. W.: Distinctions and correspondences among surfaces containing blood. *Ann. N.Y. Acad. Sci.* 516: 196-203 (1987).

[12] Baier, R. E., V. A. Depalme, D. W. Goupil, E. Cohen: Human platelet spreading on substrata of know surface chemistry. *J. Biomed. Mater. Res.* 19: 1157-1167 (1985).

[13] Kim, S. W., H. Jacobs, J. Y. Lin, C. Nojori, T. Okano: Non-thrombogenic bioactive surfaces. *Ann. N.Y. Acad. Sci.* 516: 116-130 (1987).

[14] Salzmann, E. W., J. Lindon, Ware, J. A. Mc Manama: Role of fibrinogen in activation of platelets by artificial surfaces. *Ann. N.Y. Acad. Sci.* 516: 184-195 (1987).

[15] Williams, S. K., B. E. Jarrel: Thrombosis on endothelizable surfaces. *Ann. N.Y. Acad. Sci.* 516: 145-157 (1987).

[16] Grinell, F.: Fibronectin adsorption on material surfaces. *Ann. N.Y. Acad. Sci.* 516: 280-290 (1987).

Central Venous Catheter Incompatibility and Development of a Central Register for Side Effects of Biomaterials

U. T. Seyfert, G. Pindur, C. Miyashita, G. Jutzler, R. Bambauer, E. Wenzel

Abstract

One of the most frequent complications of central venous catheters is thrombogenicity. We will report on our own observations leading to the predictivity of laboratory tests in clinical investigations or diagnosis of incompatibilities due to catheters. Attempts to realize on a national as well as international level a Central Register for documenting clinically relevant side effects will be reported in detail. Implementation of the registry involves the review of present literature and standardization procedures. An incompatibility report/questionnaire has been developed. The aims of registering and evaluating these reports will be demonstrated and discussed in detail.

Introduction

In West Germany about 1.5 million patients are treated yearly with indwelling catheters. The average intravenous time is 2.3 days. Estimated figures of central venous catheters are contamination in 5 %, sepsis in 0.5 %, and thrombogenicity in 17-70 %.

Sometimes only a retrospective analysis can characterize the very complex reactions of blood material interactions, and in these patients there is often no evident relationship between an underlying disease and the biomaterial incident.

Case Reports

First case report: A 34 year old male was admitted to the Medical Center for evaluation of remittent episodes of thromboembolism and fever of unknown origin.

History: Eight years prior to admission there was a traffic accident and he stayed over a long period of time in the Intensive Care Unit. Seven years prior to admission there was a fracture of the spine L3. Additional history obtained from the patient's medical report (Table 1) included only a moderate success of therapeutical approaches with antibiotics and anticoagulants. After bleeding

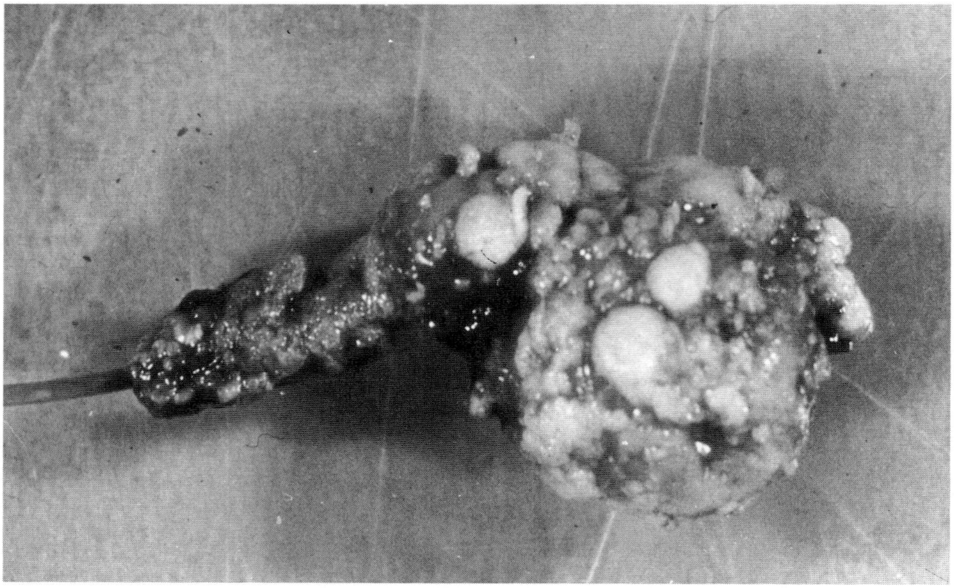

Fig. 1. Pathologic examination of a septic central venous catheter in the right ventricle.

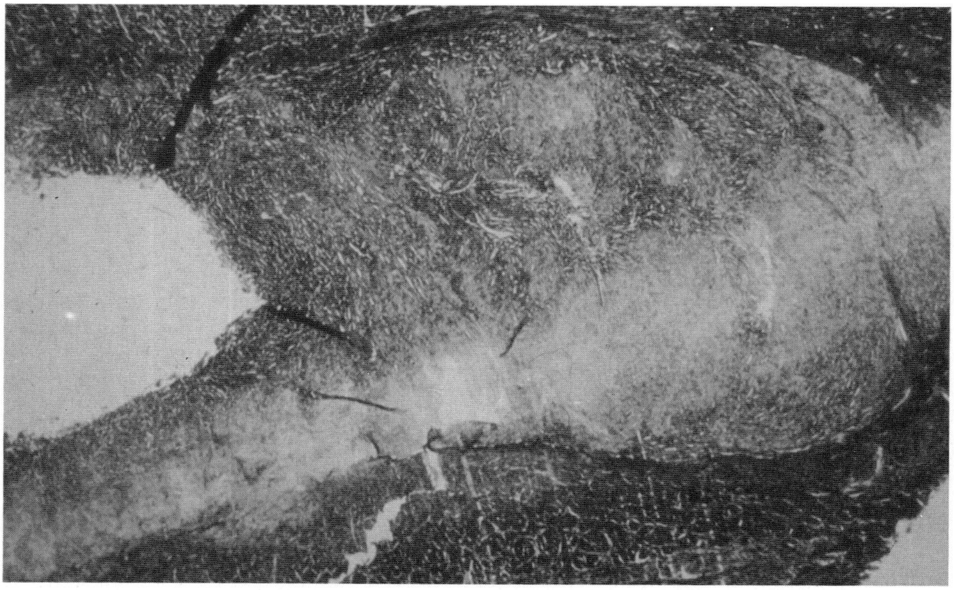

Fig. 2. Thromboembolic events due to a septic central venous catheter in the right ventricle. Pathologic examination of a vena cava superior thrombosis.

Table 1. Patient N. J. (*1952): Case report.

	Course	Complication
VII/71	Polytrauma – intensive care unit (3 w.)	contusio cerebri respiratory failure
1972/73	L 3/4 fracture	Osteomyelitis
V/72	recurrent DVT and pulmonary embolism fever of unknown origin Pseudomonas-Sepsis	thrombosis of vena cava superior bleeding complications thrombocytopenia
XII/79	Rethrombosis vena cava superior	
IX/80 +	Sepsis, pulmonary embolism, ARDS, DVT, rethrombosis vena cava superior	+ Exitus letalis

Table 2. Patient M. G. (*1932): Case report.

	Course	Complication
II/82	MI and reinfarction	arterial embolism in both legs and mesenterium Operative resection of small bowel p. o. intensive care unit: respiratory failure, acute renal failure
IV/84	Broviac catheter	cerebral embolism
V/84	aneurysmectomy and ACVB	
VII/84	venous thrombosis of Broviac catheter and vena cava superior thrombosis	
1985	MI	Exitus letalis

complications anticoagulant therapy has been disrupted and after a drop in platelet count antibiotic therapy was stopped.

In 1979 the patient was admitted to our hospital for the first time. Laboratory evaluations revealed a drop in platelet count, elevated white blood cell count, and an increased ESR. Serum creatinine and liver status in a laboratory panel were in the normal ranges. Radiographies of the chest were normal too. A sonogram of the abdomen revealed, with the exception of an increased liver and spleen size, no additional pathological findings. The patient died a few days later in the Intensive Care Unit. Sepsis and ARDS and thrombosis of the vena cava superior were the clinical findings. Pathologic examination confirmed the thromboembolic events in the lungs and upper vena cava superior due to a septic central venous catheter with thrombotic deposits in the right ventricle (Fig. 1, 2).

In 1971, eight years prior to admission, the patient's treatment included therapy with a central venous catheter.

Second case report: A 52 year old male (Table 2) was admitted in our Medical Center with severe angina pectoris. After confirming a myocardial infarction the patient developed certain complications due to an aneurysma in the infarct area. Several thromboembolic episodes appeared, e.g. in the mesenterium and resection up to 30 cm of the upper small bowel followed. Several days after discharge the patient developed a cerebral embolic episode. Though aneurysmectomy and ACVB had to be performed. The nutritional state improved after implantation of a Silastic Broviac catheter. Six months later there was a further admission to the hospital with thrombosis of the upper vena cava and typical clinical signs. In view of the patient's history he underwent radiography and thrombosis of the Broviac catheter could be confirmed.

Table 3. Hypercoaguable state.

1)	Catheter surface.
2)	Neointima.
3)	Activation of coagulation system.
4)	Disturbances in RES/RHS clearance.

Our laboratory panel revealed normal serum electrolytes, BUN, creatinine, blood, glucose, electrophoresis, urine-analysis, vitamin B 12, folic acid, and a coagulation lab panel in a normal range with the exception of a drop in the Antithrombin III activity and concentration (Fig. 3). There are certain factors contributing to the AT III deficiency (Table 3).

AT III deficiencies are not common causes of catheter thrombosis and catheter incompatibility.

A lysis therapy with urokinase was begun. We could demonstrate the safety and the efficacy of urokinase lysis therapy (Fig. 4, 5). There are certain advantages how to remove the catheter because after catheter removal lysis therapy could only be performed with a delay of time.

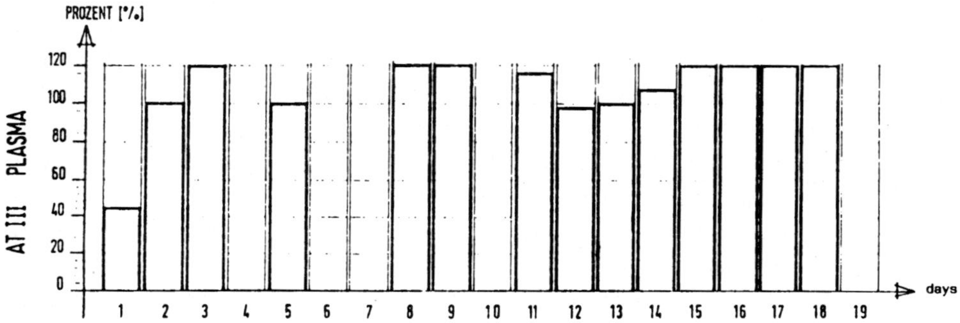

Fig. 3. Patient M.G.: Laboratory panel (I).

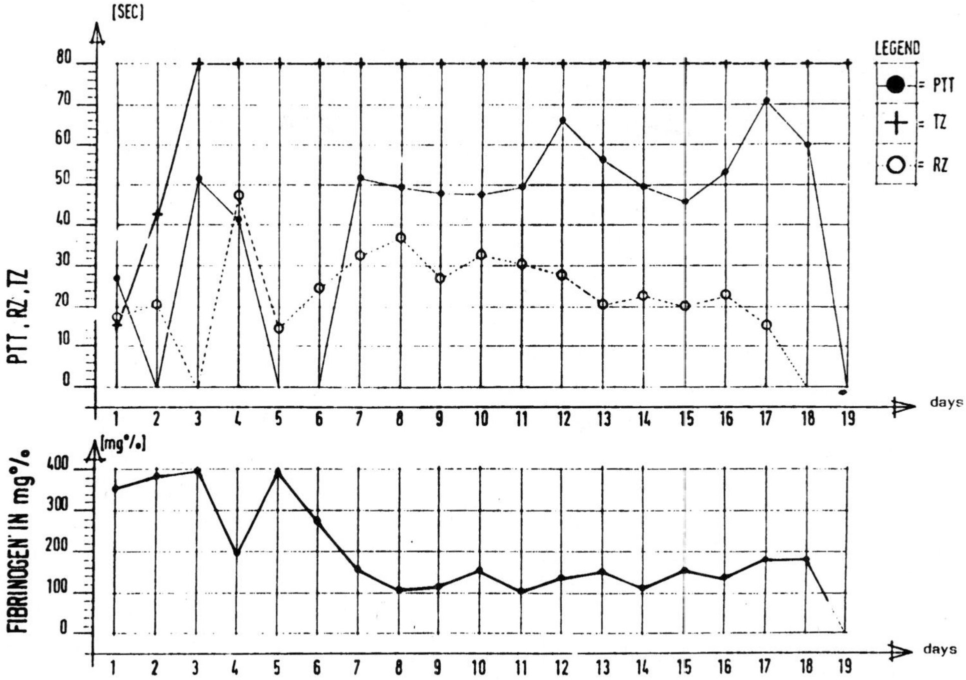

Fig. 4. Patient M.G.: Laboratory panel (II).

Discussion

The first interaction between blood and surface is evidently the adsorption of plasma proteins, e.g. coagulation factors on the surface [1-4]. Protein deposits on the surface are quickly followed by the adsorption of blood cells, such as white cells, platelets and red cells. These processes are influenced by the surface physics, the blood flow as well as the coagulation and immune defense system. According to Nosé we recognize similar alterations in human pathophysiological behavior due to foreign surface-blood incompatibilities and during allograft rejection episodes (Table 4). Therefore, only an approach using our current knowledge of human immune defense system will lead to convincing results. The use of ex vivo systems of course can differentiate and characterize interactions of polymers and surfaces, but loss of endothelium explains a wide gap between ex vivo systems and clinical relevance. With the above mentioned special hypothesis we will gain sufficient evidence of the nature of an underlying bioincompatibility process.

Obviously, the need for solving this complex problem calls for an extensive exchange of knowledge and very close cooperation between scientists from all fields involved. Thus, we need to investigate clinical aspects of biocompatibility of foreign

Table 4. Hypothesis: Interaction of polymers with living systems. Comparison with rejection episodes after allograft transplantation.

Implantation of Artificial Organs	Histology	Main Problems	Allograft Transplantation
I Confusion Stage (hours)	Vessels: necrosis, edema, fibrin, leukocyte, monocyte infiltration	red thrombus	hyperacute rejection
II Fighting Stage (< 3 weeks)	Changes in Interstitium, loss of endothelium integrity	white thrombus	acute rejection
III Live together Stage (> 3 weeks)	Calcification, pannus formation, intima fibrosis	intima fibrosis, hyalinosis	chronic rejection

materials according to the efforts undertaken in the field of pharmaceutical side effects on a national and to some extent international level.

In 1984 the Department of Biomathematics in conjunction with the Department of Haemostaseology and Transfusion Medicine at the University of Saarland, FRG, were accorded the task of establishing on an international level a Central Register for documenting clinically relevant side effects resulting from the use of biomaterial. The actual organization of the registry is listed up in the flow diagram (Table 5, 6).

Table 5. CBR-Organization I.

Central Bioincompatibility Registry (CBR)
Documentation of incident reports ⟺ references (data base)
⇒ Analysis and references (proposal) directed to scientific comitee
⇐ Output of statements
Chairmen: E. Wenzel, G. A. Jutzler Data base computer-supported ROM-C: W. Heinrich Keywords, References: St. Bohnerth Secretary: U. T. Seyfert, G. Pindur
Experimental Hemostaseology (Laboratory):
U. T. Seyfert, G. Pindur
Rheology: H. Kiesewetter Biotechnology: F. Jung
Standardization of laboratory methods and biomaterials (polymers).

A bioincompatibility incident report has been developed according to the Report on Pharmaceutical Side Effects of the "Deutsche Arzneimittelkommission der Deutschen Ärzteschaft". This incident report should contain the name of the biomaterial used, how long it was used, and also which medications were being administered. This questionnaire shall be obtainable from physician associations,

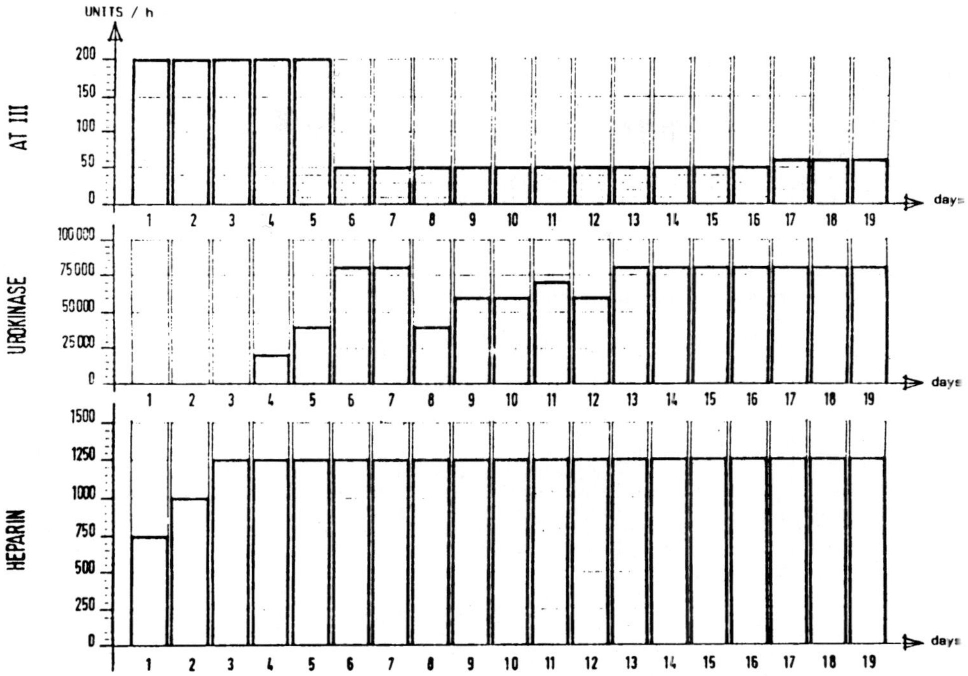

Fig. 5. Patient M.G.: Therapeutical approaches.

DAB/GTH, ICHT, and of course the Central Register at Homburg/Saar. Physician organizations are requested to publish these incident reports in their bulletins and journals. The Central Register can provide access to essential information by indicating the major categories and a number of keywords.

Bulletins with reports and editorials on the present state will be published on a half-year basis beginning 1989. The main criteria for registering and evaluation of these reports can be summarized:

1. Objective evaluation by standardization of laboratory and diagnostic methods.
2. Appointment of reference laboratories and submitting of proposed and tentative standards.
3. Differentiation between toxicity, blood and tissue incompatibility.
4. Relationship of biomaterial to physical-chemical basis of the biomaterial device.
5. Interaction of flow characteristics and bioincompatibility specific devices.
6. Characterization of clinical aspects of biomaterial incompatibility.
7. Statistical evaluation of frequency, clinical intensity and duration of side effects
8. Incidence of side effects with or without use of biomaterial.
9. Interaction with medication and specific pharmaceutical agents or therapeutic methods.
10. Convenient access to information in the data bank of the Central Register.

Table 6. CBR-Organization II.

Universitätskliniken im Saarland		
↓	↓	
Department of Hemodialysis and Nephrology	Department of Clinical Hemostaseology and Transfusion Medicine	Exp. laboratory work (biocompatibility testing)
↓	↓	↓
Central Bioincompatibility Registry (CBR)		Scientific Organization (and official medical bodies)
Documentation of reports	Data base of references	Biomedical research and industrial production
↓	↕	....
Scientific Comitee	Arzneimittelkommission der Deutschen Ärzteschaft	....
Chairmen:	Registry of Pace makers	
G. A. Jutzler, Homburg/S.	Registry of artificial lents	
Y. Nosé, Cleveland	....	
E. Wenzel, Homburg/Saar	....	
....		
....		

Conclusions

The immediate and ultimate goal of the Central Register is prompt recognition of unexpected side effects and evaluation of biomaterials. This can only be achieved by intensified national and international collaboration.

References

[1] FISCHER, J. P., P. FUHGE, K. BURG, N. HEIMBURGER: Methoden zur Herstellung und Charakterisierung von Kunststoffen mit verbesserter Blutverträglichkeit. *Die Angewandte Makromolekulare Chemie* 105: 131-165 (1982).

[2] PELZER, H.: Biochemical methods to evaluate blood compatibility of biomaterials. In: PLANCK, H., G. EGBERS, I. SYRE (eds.): Polyurethanes in Biomedical Engineering, pp. 69-81, 1984.

[3] WENZEL, E., M. KÖHLER, P. HELLSTERN, G. HARBAUER, J. VOLKMER, R. KRÜGER: Zur Prüfung und Charakterisierung der Blutverträglichkeit von körperfremden Oberflächen. In: Verhandlungsber. d. 25. Tagung d. Dt. Arbeitsgemeinschaft f. Blutgerinnungsforschung, pp. 165-350, 1982.

[4] YOUNG, B. R., L. K. LAMBRECHT, S. L. COOPER, D. F. MOSHER: Plasma proteins: Their role in initiating platelet and fibrin deposition on biomaterials. In: COOPER, S. L. (ed.): Biomaterials: interfacial phenomena and applications, Adv. Chem. Series Washington D. C., pp. 317-350, 1982.

Catheter Technology: Techniques

Techniques for Percutaneous Puncturing of Large Vessels

R. Bambauer

Abstract

Since the introduction of large bore catheters for acute hemodialysis, 30 years ago, a large number of problems with handling, material and contamination of these catheters were existent.

Nevertheless the catheterization of the cava inferior and superior with large bore catheters has proven to be suitable as a rapid connection process for hemodialysis, hemofiltration, hemoperfusion, plasmapheresis, plasmaperfusion, etc.

Besides the different puncture techniques, the side effects and complications in our own observation are described and compared with the literature.

Introduction

In 1979 when I was assigned to the Department of Nephrology of the University of Saarland, I quickly became aware of the problems associated with vascular access points in patients suffering from end stage renal disease (ESRD). Therefore, I introduced, in early 1979, percutaneous puncturing of the internal jugular vein (int. jug. vein) and the placing of a large bore catheter applying the Seldinger technique [1, 2].

The first catheter was positioned in a 17 years old male patient suffering from acute exacerbation associated with chronic renal insufficiency and extreme hyperhydration who was in a very poor condition and required acute dialysis. Compelled to treat the boy, we took the risk without realizing what we were letting ourselves in for. Without any considerable problem we were able, to find the int. jug. vein, using the Seldinger technique, to introduce a large bore catheter. The boy was then dialysed, and recompensated by regular dialysis treatments. This all happened not quite ten years ago. We are still looking after this patient.

From this point onwards we often had the opportunity of applying this catheter technique and established this procedure in our Department. In subsequent years catheter technology proved to be an enormous gain for the dialysis technique and surely represents one of the most important steps forward made over the last few years. Herein we will limit ourselves to puncturing techniques, catheter localization and hygienic measures.

Shunt problems are often encountered during acute and chronic hemodialysis treatment and even temporary vascular access such as the Scribner shunt and femoral catheter also involve considerable problems. Therefore many physicians have, over the last few years, introduced catheterization of the vena cava superior using a large bore catheter [3-12].

As early as 1961 Shaldon et al. described the possibility of percutaneously catheterization of the femoral artery and vein for hemodialysis treatment [13]. Over the following years these methods were almost exclusively used as temporary access points for acute dialysis, as the peripheral extremity vessels were preserved in case of vascular anastomosis at a later date. Before long only the femoral vein was percutaneously punctured [13-18]. However, catheterization of the femoral vein carried a 4 % risk of lethal complications. Schwarzbeck therefore described in 1979 catheterization of the vena cava superior over the subclavian vein [3, 4]. The possibilities of catheterization of the vena cava inferior and superior for insertion of large bore catheters are shown in Table 1.

Table 1. Catherization of vena cava inferior and superior for insertion of large bore catheters.

1961	Shaldon et al.	A. / V. femoralis	[13]
1963	Shaldon et al.	A. / V. femoralis	[14]
1975	Kjellstrand et al.	V. femoralis	[15]
1977	Fuchs et al.	V. femoralis	[16]
1977	Kramer et al.	A. / V. femoralis	[17]
1979	Lederle et al.	V. femoralis	[18]
1978	Schwarzbeck et al.	V. subclavia	[3]
1978	De Cubber	V. subclavia	[5]
1978	Hennemann	V. subclavia	[6]
1979	Uldall et al.	V. subclavia	[7]
1980	Uldall et al.	V. subclavia	[8]
1980	Leb	V. subclavia	[9]
1980	Flynn et al.	V. subclavia	[10]
1981	Uldall et al.	V. subclavia	[11]
1983	Taylor et al.	V. subclavia	[12]
1979	Bambauer et al.	V. jugularis interna	[1]
1981	Spiegel	V. sub. / V. jugularis interna	[19]
1982	Bambauer et al.	V. jugularis interna	[20, 21]

Catheter and Material

The large bore catheter has been frequently modified over recent years and all models available are of a similar construction. With an inner diameter of between 1.5 and 1.8 mm they are available in lengths of 80 to 200 mm. The tip terminates in a cone and is usually of 0.8 mm diameter. On the side of the catheter, depending on the model, 6-12 perforations are found, on the one hand, to guarantee more effective blood flow and on the other hand to prevent the catheter from adhering to the vascular wall. The clinical tip allows easier introduction of the catheter and prevents thrombi forming in the bore and passing through to the blood stream. Now the various catheter models also have an inner catheter which can be inserted under sterile conditions after each hemodialysis treatment and left in place until the next extracorporeal treatment. These inner catheters close the catheter bore and thus prevent the intraluminal formation of thrombi. In addition to this it provides additional security between treatments (Fig. 1).

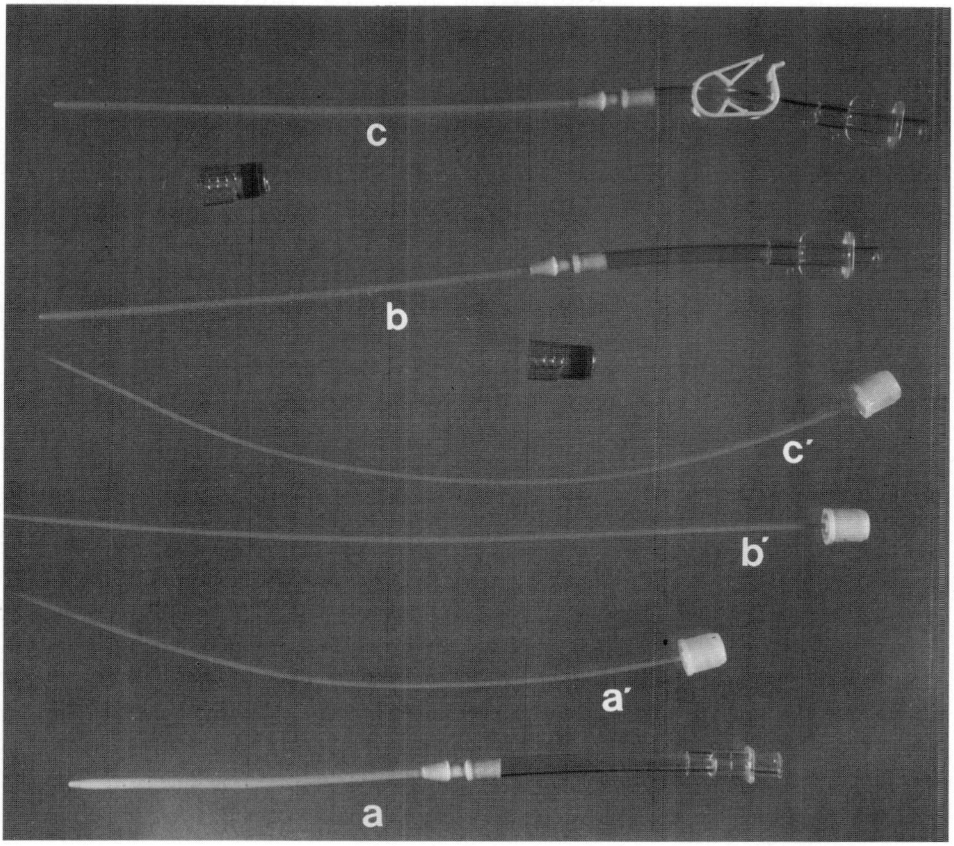

Fig. 1. Large bore and inner catheters with different lengths (a: 100 mm, b: 140 mm, c: 150 mm; a', b', c': inner catheters; Bellco, Mirandola, Italy).

Catheters which became available over the last few years still, in some cases, had considerable defects such as, for example, sharp edged tips, too rigid material, uneven transitions from catheter to the silicone tube connection and insufficiently adhering luer lock connectors. These defects caused at times considerable complications, making new developments necessary [22].

Teflon catheters have a very smooth surface and thus a low thrombogenity. Other catheters are made of polyurethane which has also proved to be of good biocompatibility and low thrombogenity. This material is somewhat more elastic than Teflon. Polypropylene is used as catheter material but its rough surface must be siliconized before use. Silicone catheters positioned by surgical implant techniques also have a good tissue compatibility (Table 2).

Table 2. Advantages and disadvantages of different catheter materials.

Catheter Material	Advantage	Disadvantage
Teflon	smooth surface, low thrombogenity	not elastic enough, SEM* : surface is rigid, long longitudinal axis
Polyurethane	good biocompatibility, low thrombogenity, very elastic, SEM: very smooth surface	–
Polypropylene	with siliconized surface, low thrombogenity	not enough elastic, SEM: surfaces were very uneven and contained many small pits
Silicone	good biocompatibility	–

* SEM : Scanning Electron Microscopy

Not all commercially available catheters provide a contrasted picture when x-rayed. The incorporation of contrast medium presents no problem with polyurethane catheters while with Teflon material this may affect the durability of the material. Initially this leads to the catheter breaking at points where it is mechanically particularly stressed [12]. Further development has resolved this problem but these catheters now have somewhat thicker walls. This can, however, lead to increased irritation of the endothelium. Catheters providing contrast are not absolutely necessary as the position can be controlled more simply and gently with an intraatrial ECG lead [23-28]. It is of decisive importance that the catheter material is well tolerated and of low thrombosity.

Method

Puncturing must always be carried out under aseptic conditions, (i.e. through, extensive cleaning of the puncture area, disinfection, sterile drapes and gowns, masks, surgical gloves, etc.). The patient should be correctly positioned according to the vascular access point to be used and should be given adequate local anaesthetic [10].

The vena cava inferior and vena cava superior are particularly suitable as central vascular access points. The vena cava inferior is reached by puncturing the femoral vein and placing the catheter. If the catheter remains in place for a longer period there is a risk of potentially lethal complications such as bacterial infections and thromboembolism. Although the complication rate is low for catheters which remain only a short time in position or if they are removed after each hemodialysis treatment, this puncture technique should only be used for particular indications.

The vena cava superior can be reached in a variety of ways over the internal jugular vein and the subclavian vein. Here too for each vascular access point there are different puncturing locations. Each location has advantages and disadvantages. which usually depend on the dexterity of the treating physician.

With the puncturing technique used for the vena subclavia it is often difficult to guide the large bore catheter beneath the clavicule. Due to the anatomical position of the subclavian vein it is more likely that the large bore catheter causes a perforation, in addition to the danger of inducing a pneumothorax or hematothorax If the catheter remains in position over a longer period endothelial lesions in the vein wall are very likely as the catheter, because of its rigidness, may stretch the vessel [6].

As previously mentioned, we prefer to use the internal jugular vein, as it runs in an almost straight line from the base of the skull in the immediate vicinity of the arteria leading to the truncus brachiocephalicus. The lower part is found subcutaneously between the caputs of the musculus sternocleidomastoideus. The right internal jugular vein is the shortest connection to the right atrium and is therefore particularly suitable for percutaneous puncture [29-31]. If the guidelines set down by the puncture technique are observed a skilled physician is able to successfully execute puncture, 90 % at the first attempt [20, 21].

If the catheter remains in position over a longer period bacteria may invade the length of the penetration channel of the catheter lumen. It is therefore often appropriate for both subclavian and internal jugular vein punctures to tunnel the catheter subcutaneously over a distance of 2-5 cm.

Before fixing the catheter with a suture, its position and particularly that of the catheter tip should be checked. Many catheters are contrasted on x-ray pictures which means that catheter position can be checked with a thorax x-ray. However, as a normal radiological control with x-ray film or image converter takes time and requires extensive apparatus, in addition to which the patient is exposed to radiation, we apply the ECG lead to the large bore catheter [32, 33].

Initially the tip of the catheter was localized with T-shaped metal pieces which were attached to the catheter but we now use a J-guide [34]. A metal wire, covered with plastic is situated up to the bend of the J-guide (Fig. 2). Once introduced the J-guide can be positioned by a slight to and for movement so that the bent tip catches on to the catheter tip and the intraatrial ECG lead thus actually originates from the catheter tip. As most catheter models have 6-12 perforations along the side at distances of 3-5 cm from the catheter tip, theoretically an intraatrial ECG could also be fed out of the first perforation over a blood column or fluid column.

The J-guide however, makes the localization of the catheter tip possible. Figure 3 shows the intraatrial ECG. The catheter should be placed in a cava superior position.

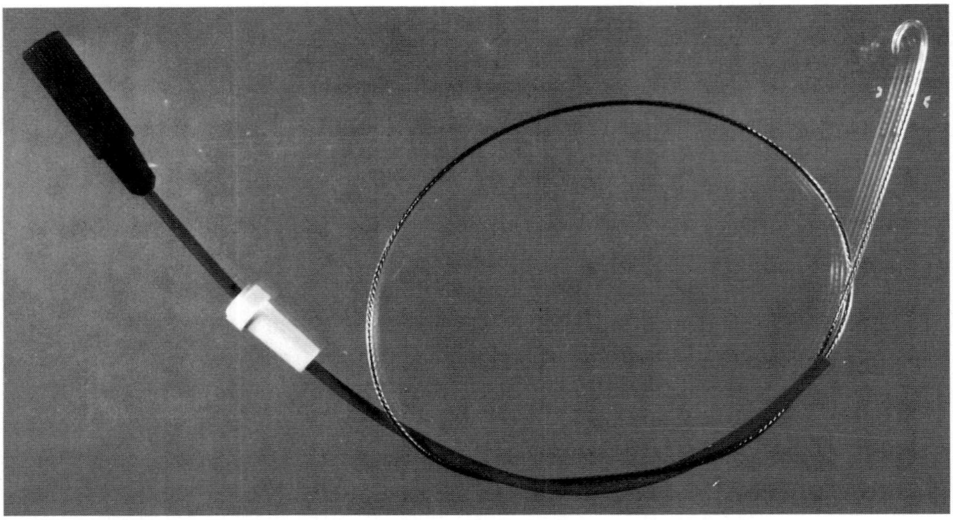

Fig. 2. J-guide for introducing the large bore catheter and leading an intraarterial ECG. ⇒ : The metal wire which ends here, is covered with plastic. The introduced J-Guide can be positioned so that the bent tip catches on the catheter tip (J-Guide, Sterimed, Saarbrücken, FRG).

Percutaneous puncturing of a central venous vessel and the laying of a large bore catheter is not without complications and therefore requires careful assessment of the indications. The primary puncture risk depends first and foremost on the dexterity and experience of the physician. Subsequent complications usually depend on the time the catheter remains in position. It is therefore difficult to compare the results presented to date.

Results

With the help of a few results a list of complications can be drawn up and, in as far as this is possible, compared to results published in literature. The primary risk for the femoral vein is very low. However, Burri et al. in 1976 presented results which showed that if a vein catheter remained in position in the femoral vein for a longer period quite a high complication rate was observed [35]. Infections involving phlebitis and/or sepsis lead to a mortality of 4 %, a short in-dwelling time of 2-3 days or regular removal after each treatment, as described by Kjellstrand and

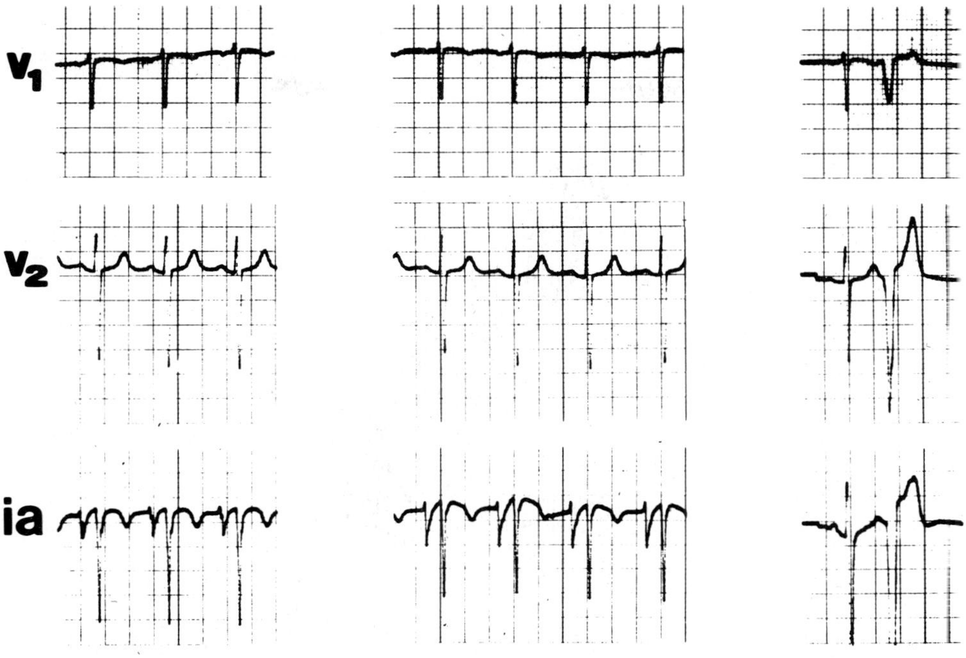

Fig. 3. Intraaterial ECG. The catheter should be placed in a cave superior position.

Küppers et al. usually avoids complications but means higher traumatism of the femoral vessels [15, 51].

The Table 3 sets out our own complication rates for different central vein access points [37] compared to those of Schwarzbeck [52]. Schwarzbeck gives a complication rate of over 70 % for puncture of the internal jugular vein, while we only experienced complications in 21.5 % of our patients [52]. The complication rates for puncture of the subclavian and femoral veins are fairly similar. From the number of punctures carried out it can clearly be seen that some vessels are preferred to others.

Infections have been listed in second position, the most severe complication here is a so-called catheter sepsis. Every catheter sepsis can have severe consequences for the patient, and for this reason under these conditions the catheter should be removed and antibiotic therapy started immediately.

In order to stop the risk of infection, that is to say the invasion of bacteria caused by incorrect handling of the catheter, we have developed a protection against contamination, which will become available within the next few months (Fig. 4). After each dialysis an inner catheter with this contamination safeguard will be

Table 3. Complication rates by puncturing of large vessels for insertion of large bore catheters.

Complications	Schwarzbeck 1983 [52]			Bambauer 1984 [37]		
	V. jug. (n = 155) %	V. sub. (n = 674) %	V.fem. (n = 278) %	V. jug. (n = 727) %	V. sub. (n = 166) %	V.fem. (n = 7) %
Faulty puncture						
– Puncture of artery	29.6	2.5	9.0	3.2	0.6	–
Infections						
– Puncture site	13.9	12.0	1.4	3.3	5.4	–
– Abscess	6.0	11.8	8.3	1.2	3.6	14.3
– Sepsis	9.6	2.8	0.7	1.8	7.2	–
Thrombosis						
– V. jug.	–	–	–	0.3	–	–
– V. sub.	–	0.15	–	–	4.8	–
Miscellaneous						
– Bleeding	6.7	1.9	6.2	1.0	2.4	–
– Hematothorax	–	1.15	–	–	0.6	–
– Pneumothorax	–	0.7	–	–	2.4	–
– Embolism	–	0.75	–	–	–	–
– Pain	1.7	0.7	1.4	–	–	–
Faulty catheter material	10.3	11.8	1.6	8.9	9.0	14.3
Total	77.3	45.35	28.6	21.5	38.4	28.6

V. jug.: V. jugularis; V. sub.: V. subclavia; V. fem.: V. femoralis.

positioned, under sterile conditions, and left in place until the next hemodialysis. Current results have shown that the risk of infection and bacterial population were clearly reduced if this contamination safeguard is used (Table 4).

Another complication on the Table 3 is thrombosis. However, the catheter terminating in a cone was a decisive advantage because the thromboses forming intraluminally could not be conveyed to the heart. We have been closing large bore catheters between extracorporeal treatments with an inner catheter for over four years. Extensive thrombosing around the catheter or initiating from the catheter without completely closing the lumen was observed with internal jugular catheters. In a small number of subclavian catheters thromboses were diagnosed on one or both subclavian veins angiographically or in an autopsy.

Bleeding or after bleeding is slight for internal jugular vein and subclavian vein punctures, sufficient compression brings most bleeding to a halt unless the patient suffers from a considerable coagulation disorder. Other complications observed are hematothorax, pneumothorax and misplacements, particularly with subclavian catheters.

Damaged catheter material is not inconsiderable, but is mostly caused by incorrect handling. However, catheters are now available which no longer have the initial problems such as breaking off of individual parts, cracks, kinks and similar.

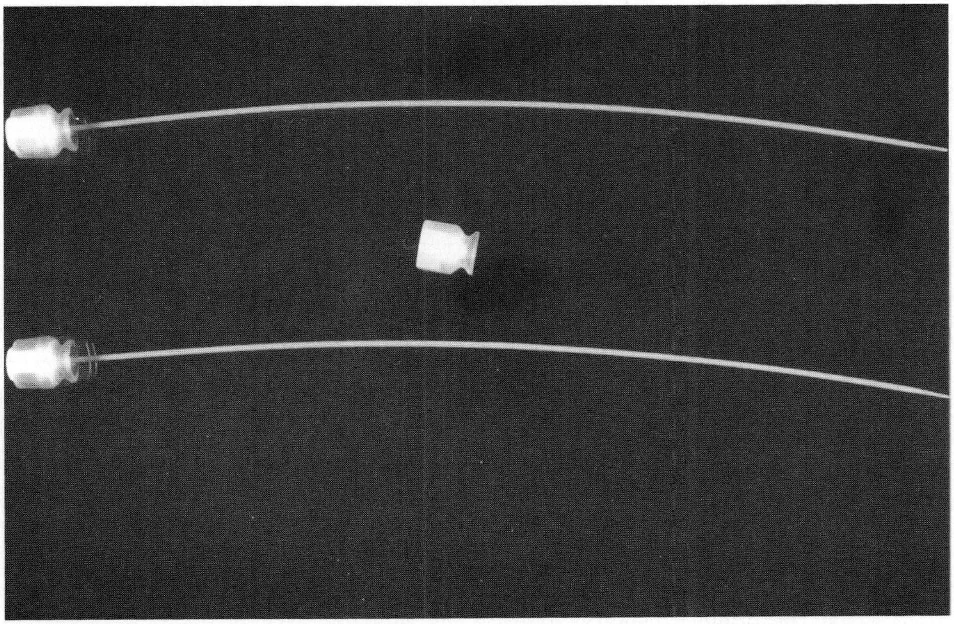

Fig. 4. Inner catheter with contamination safeguard (Inner catheter: Bellco, Mirandola, Italy; Contamination Safeguard: Sterimed, Saarbrücken, FRG).

Discussion

The following conclusions can be drawn from the above exposition [30, 34, 36, 38-44]: access over the internal jugular vein appears to be the safest way to the vena cava superior due to the much lower complication rate and the good puncturing position. It is thus clearly better than puncturing the femoralis and subclavian veins. The most commonly observed complication is the puncture of the arteria carotis [35]. The bleeding can, however, quickly be stopped with compression for 5-6 minutes. In this connection cerebrovascular complications leading to death after mispuncture have also been described [45-50].

One of the reasons for faulty puncturing worth mentioning is that often too thick and too long puncture canulae are used, and some hyperhydrated patients, because of breathlessness, cannot be correctly positioned and others because of their acute condition are often restless and confused. In these cases, if the physician is less experienced, puncture with a thin needle with the help of a sonograph is recommended.

An important factor for causing thrombosis is the extent to which the vein wall is traumatised. Every puncture causes wall hematoma to a greater or lesser degree and if these hematoma are continually touched they become considerably enlarged,

Table 4. Bacteriological results with a contamination safeguard in large bore catheters.

Pat. No.	Catheter in situ (days)	HD / TPE (n)	Contamination safeguard (n)	Bacteriological results			
				inner surface		outer surface	
				neg.	pos.	neg.	pos.
1	141	60 HD	21	6	15	20	1
2	84	39 HD	9	3	6	8	1
3	74	39 HD	10	4	6	9	1
4	51	42 HD/ 10 TPE	29	9	20	26	3
5	28	9 TPE	8	4	4	8	–
6	95	73 HD / 18 TPE	20	5	15	20	–
7	117	52 HD	25	10	15	24	1
8	89	27 HD	28	4	24	28	–
9	58	20 HD	13	4	9	13	–
10	38	13 HD	9	4	5	8	1
11	64	22 HD	8	2	6	8	–
		Total	180	55	125 (69.4%)	172	8 (4.4%)

turning into perivascular hematoma and then to thrombosis [49]. Therefore it follows that the puncture should damage the vessel as little as possible. A skilled physician is able to successfully puncture the vein at the first attempt in more than 90 % of the cases.

The introduction of the catheter under sterile conditions and solicitous nursing is of outmost importance after disinfection of the skin. It is also advisable to use contamination safeguards under sterile conditions (Fig. 4). Bandages must be renewed every second or third day, skin smears for bacteriological examination should be taken regularly. Prophylactic administration of antibiotics is not necessary. In particularly weak patients the catheter should be tunneled through 2-5 cm of skin.

It is necessary to localize the position of the catheter and its tip after each catheterization of the vena cava superior with a large bore catheter. This can be done with a radiological image of the catheter or particularly effectively with an intraatrial electrocardiogram. The latter method is more simple and quicker to implement, misplacement can be more quickly detected and corrected and the patient is not exposed to radiation.

However, it must be said that percutaneous positioning of large bore catheters in central venous vessels has greatly simplified acute extracorporeal detoxication measures and allows more rapid execution. Percutaneous puncturing of the internal jugular vein and subclavia for catheterizing the vena cava superior has proved to be a highly suitable and quickly applicable method of connection for hemodialysis, hemofiltration and hemoperfusion, plasmapheresis and plasma perfusion. This procedure has proved to be the most rapid and free of complications, particularly for acute treatment such as, for example, exogenous intoxications, hyperhydration, lung edemas, severe electrolyte dysfunctions, and hemodilution after heart operations.

A few minutes after indication a large catheter can be laid and treatment started with the single needle technique. The introduction of catheterization with a large bore catheter has, at least in our Department, made the previously necessary use of a Scribner shunt superfluous. Puncturing of the internal jugular vein and vena subclavia as temporary vascular access point are adequate in almost all situations although we prefer to puncture the internal jugular vein because of the lower complication rate and the better puncturing possibility.

Contraindication for internal jugular vein catheterization are only inflammations at the point of puncture and unidentified anatomical conditions, e.g. extended strumae or tumors in the neck area.

References

[1] BAMBAUER, R., G. A. JUTZLER: Shaldon-Katheterisierung über die V. Jugularis interna, ein neuer Zugang für akute Hämodialyse. *Nieren- und Hochdruckkrankh.* 8: 218 (1979).

[2] BAMBAUER, R., G. A. JUTZLER: Jugularis-interna-Punktion zur Shaldon-Katheterisierung. Ein neuer Zugang für akute Hämodialysen. *Nieren- und Hochdruckkrankh.* 9: 109 (1980).

[3] SCHWARZBECK, A., W.-D. BRITTINGER, G. E. VON HENNING, M. STRAUCH: Cannulation of subclavian vein for hemodialysis using Seldinger's technique. *Trans. Am. Soc. Artif. Intern. Org.* 27 (1978).

[4] SCHWARZBECK, A., W.-D. BRITTINGER: Erfahrungen mit großlumigen Venenkathetern zur Akuthämodialyse. *Prakt. Anästh.* 13: 102 (1978).

[5] CUBBER, A. DE, C. DE WOLF, N. LAMEIRE, M. SCHURGERS, S. RINGOIR: Single-needle hemodialysis with the double headpump via the subclavian vein. *Dial. Transpl.* 7: 1261 (1978).

[6] HENNEMANN, H.: Die Vena subclavia - Akutdialysezugang der ersten Wahl? *Intensivmedizin* 15: 236 (1978).

[7] ULDALL, P. R., R. F. DYCK, F. WOODS, N. MERCHANT, G. S. MARTIN, C. J. CARDELLA, D. M. C. SUTTON: A subclavian cannula for temporary vascular access for hemodialysis or plasmapheresis. *Dial. Transpl.* 8: 963 (1979).

[8] ULDALL, P. R., F. WOODS, N. MERCHANT: A double-lumen subclavian cannula (DLSC) for temporary haemodialysis access. *ASAIO Abstracts* 9: 38 (1980).

[9] LEB, D. E.: An introduction to hemodialysis renal nursing symposium: Part II. *Dial. Transpl.* 9: 571 (1980).

[10] FLYNN, C. T., R. MC GOWAN: Subclavian vein catheter and clockwork pump. *Dial. Transpl.* 9: 556 (1980).

[11] ULDALL, P. R., P. WILLIAMS: The subclavian cannula: Temporary vascular access for hemodialysis when long-term peritoneal dialysis has to be interrupted. *Peritoneal Dial. Bull.* 1: 97 (1981).

[12] TAYLOR, G., J. M. BONE: A new silastic subclavian cannula for hemodialysis or plasma exchange. *Dial. Transpl.* 12: 26 (1983).

[13] SHALDON, S., L. CHIANDUSSI, B. HIGGS: Haemodialysis by percutaneous catheterization of the femoral artery and vein with regional heparinization. *Lancet* II: 857 (1961).

[14] SHALDON, S., A. I. RAE, S. M. ROSEN, H. SILVA, J. OAKLEY: Refrigerated femoral venous-venous haemodialysis with coil preservation for rehabilitation of terminal uraemic patients. *Br. Med. J.* 1: 1716 (1963).

[15] KJELLSTRAND, C. M., G. E. MERINO, S. M. MAUER, R. CASALI, T. J. BUSELMEIER: Complications of percutaneous femoral vein catheterizations for hemodialysis. *Clin. Nephrol.* 4: 37 (1975).

[16] FUCHS, H. J., G. JENETT, U. KLEHR, G. RICHTER, R. WILBRANDT, U. FROTSCHER: Die perkutane Punktion der Vena femoralis zur Hämodialysebehandlung. *Dtsch. Med. Wochenschr.* 102: 1280 (1977).

[17] KRAMER, P., C. LANGENSCHEID, D. MATTHEI, J. RIEGER: Behandlung der Diuretika-resistenten Überwässerung mit arteriovenöser Hämofiltration. In: SCHELER, F. VON, H. V. HENNING (eds.): Hämofiltration. Dustri-Verlag, Dr. Karl Feistle, München-Deisenhofen, pp. 23-28 (1977).

[18] LEDERLE, R. M., H. J. PORTMANN, G. WERMUTH: Erfahrungen mit einem modifizierten Femoral-Katheter zur Hämodialyse-Behandlung. *Intensivmedizin* 16: 258 (1979).

[19] SPIEGEL, P., R. PILGRIM, U. GESSLER: Die Bedeutung großlumiger Venenkatheter für extrakorporale Eliminationsverfahren in der Intensivtherapie. *Intensivmedizin* 18: 301 (1981).

[20] BAMBAUER, R., G. A. JUTZLER: Erfahrungen mit großlumigen Verweilkathetern in der V. jugularis interna als Zugang für akute Hämodialysen. *Klin. Wochenschr.* 60: 285 (1982).

[21] BAMBAUER, R., G. A. JUTZLER: Transcutaneous insertion of the Shaldon catheter through the internal jugular vein as access for acute hemodialysis. *Dial. Transpl.* 11: 766 (1982).

[22] BAMBAUER, R.: Therapeutischer Plasmaaustausch und verwandte Plasmaseparationsverfahren. Technische Grundlagen, Pathophysiologie und klinische Ergebnisse. Schattauer : Stuttgart-New York, 1988.

[23] GÖTZ, E.: Stellungnahme zum Beitrag von F. J. Loers: Erfahrungen mit dem intrakardialen EKG zur Lagekontrolle des Cava-Katheters. *Anästhesiol. Intensivmed.* 20: 68 (1979).

[24] HUFNAGL, H. D., S. SEN, M. SCHERZER, G. RETTIG: Intraatriale EKG-Diagnostik über Cava-Katheter. *Intensivmedizin* 12: 433 (1975).

[25] KLINNERT, U.: Transvenöse Elektrodenkatheter als Hilfsmittel zur Diagnostik. *Diagnostik* 10: 127 (1977).

[26] LOERS, F. J.: Klinische Erfahrungen mit dem Kavakatheter über die Vena jugularis interna. *Prakt. Anästh.* 11: 28 (1976).

[27] NIEMAN, W., D. KOCH: Lagebestimmung zentralvenöser Katheter durch intrakardiale EKG-Ableitung. *Prakt. Anästh.* 11: 31 (1976).

[28] URTHALER, F., J. HALTER: Central venous catheter used for recording intracardiac electrocardiogram. A safe and reliable method for registering atrial potentials using a new device connected to the central venous catheter. *Br. Heart J.* 33: 275 (1971).

[29] DEFALQUE, R. J., B. WITTIG: Punktion und Katheterisierung der Vena jugularis interna. *Anaesthesist* 23: 41 (1973).

[30] DAILY, P. O., R. B. GRIEPP, N. E. SHUMWAY, S. CALIF: Percutaneous internal jugular vein cannulation. *Arch. Surg.* 101: 534 (1970).

[31] ENGLISH, J. C. W., R. M. FREW, J. F. PIGOTT, M. ZAKI: Percutaneous catheterization of the internal jugular vein. *Anaesthesia* 24: 521 (1969).

[32] BAMBAUER, R., G. A. JUTZLER: Lagekontrolle großlumiger zentraler Venenkatheter mittels intrakardialer Elektrokardiographie. *Intensivmedizin* 17: 317 (1980).

[33] BAMBAUER, R., G. A. JUTZLER: Use of large-bore catheters in the internal jugular vein as an access route for emergency hemodialysis. *Netherlands J. Surg.* 35: 178 (1983).

[34] JERNIGAN, W. R., W. C. GARDNER, M. M. MAHR, J. L. MILBURN: Use of the internal jugular vein for placement of central venous catheter. *Surg. Gyn. Obst.* 520 (1970).

[35] BURRI, C., G. KRISCHAK: Technik und Gefahren des Kava-Katheters. *Infusionstherapie* 3: 174 (1976).

[36] DEFALQUE, R. J.: Percutaneous catheterization of the internal jugular vein. *Anesth. Analg.* 53: 116 (1974).

[37] BAMBAUER, R.: Therapeutischer Plasmaaustausch (TPE). Untersuchungen zur Verbesserung der Anwendungstechnik, zur Kinetik, zur Erprobung neuer Membranen und der selektiven

Plasmaseparation (SPS) sowie klinische Beobachtungen. Habilitationsschrift, Med. Fakultät der Universität des Saarlandes, 1985.

[38] BURRI, C., H. HENKEMEYER, H. H. PÄSSLER: Katheterembolien. *Schweiz. Med. Wochenschr.* 101: 1537 (1971).

[39] ENGLISH, J. C. W., R. M. FREW, J. F. PIGOTT, M. ZAKI: Percutaneous central venous catheterization. Low technique: central approach. In: ROSEN, M, J. P. LATTO, W. SHANG (eds.): Handbook of percutaneous central venous catheterization. W. B. Saunders, London, Philadelphia, Toronto, pp. 98-99 (1981).

[40] FASSOLT, A., O. SCHAEFLER, U. BRAUN: Fehler und Gefahren: Medikamentöse Maßnahmen gegen Begleitthrombosen bei Cavakathetern. *Anaesthesist* 22: 224 (1973).

[41] GRANDINS, J., W. DUBEN, G. POPP: Thrombose beim Kavakatheter. *Zbl. Chir.* 98: 274-279, (1973).

[42] GRANDINS, J., G. POPP, W. DUBEN: Thrombose-Prophylaxe beim Kavakatheter. *Zbl. Chir.* 98: 280-282, (1973).

[43] HEITMAN, D., H. GRIMM, D. GASSER: Die Punktion der Vena jugularis interna, ein neuer Zugangsweg zur Vena cava superior. *Anästh. Inform.* 14: 67 (1973).

[44] HEITMAN, D., G. REGLER: Die Vena jugularis interna als Zugangsweg für den Cava-Katheter. *Klinikarzt* 5: 331 (1976).

[45] ANAGNOU, J.: Cerebrovascular accident during percutaneous cannulation of internal jugular vein (letter). *Lancet* I: 377 (1982).

[46] MC GOON, M. D., P. BENEDETTO, B. M. GREEN: Complications of percutaneous central venous catheterization: A report of two cases and review of the literature. *John Hopkins Med. J.* 145: 1 (1976).

[47] SCHWARZ, A. J., D. R. JEBES, D. R. GREENHOW, L. W. STEPHENSEN, N. ELLISON: Carotid artery puncture with internal jugular cannulation. *Anesthesiology* 51: 160 (1979).

[48] SINGBARTL, G., J. J. EISENLOHR: Hemisyndrome nach mißglückter Vena-jugularis-interna-Punktion. *Anaesthesist* 31: 95 (1982).

[49] SOLD, M., W. DÜSEL: Zerebraler Insult beim Legen eines Vena jugularis interna- Katheters. *Anaesth. Intensivther. Notfallmed.* 16: 285 (1981).

[50] WEINSCHÜTZ, W.: Arteria-cerebri-media-Verschluß nach vergeblicher Vena-jugularis-interna-Punktion. *Anaesthesist* 31: 359 (1982).

[51] KÜPPERS, H., T. RISLER, A. KRIAN, T. KÖNIGSHAUSEN, K. HOFMANN, E. SCHNUR, B. GRABENSEE: Perkutaner Zugang zu den Femoralgefäßen mittels Seldinger Technik bei der Akutdialyse. *Nieren- und Hochdruckkrankh.* 1: 43 (1976).

[52] SCHWARZBECK, A.: Möglichkeiten des temporären Gefäßzugangs. *Mitt. Klin. Nephrologie* XII: 65 (1983).

First Experience with the Percutaneous Placement of Silastic Atrium Catheters for the Short-Term Vascular Access for Hemodialysis

G. KRÖNUNG

Abstract

A technique is demonstrated in detail to place smooth Silastic catheters percutaneously. The implantation can be performed in local anesthesia by the nephrologist in the dialysis department.

In 62 cases of catheter placements no serious complication could be seen: no pneumothorax, no bleeding. Up to now no infection was noticed within function rates from one month to 24 months, but four thromboses were noted after 2-6 months. The catheter function was concordant to the good results of these Silastic catheters implanted by vasotomy.

In summary the technique of percutaneous catheter implantation presents a step forward to simplify short- and middle-term vascular access for hemodialysis, which can be performed by the nephrologist himself.

Introduction

Longer time of functioning, better handling, full mobilisation of the patient, less mechanical alteration of the vessel-wall and less discomfort for the patient enable smooth central-venous catheters to become more and more in use for the short and medium term vascular access for hemodialysis. The only disadvantage so far was the necessity to place these catheters by vasotomiam. A new technique is introduced herein which enables the percutaneous placement by the Seldinger technique and a special peel-away set (Fig. 1).

Material and Methods

When local anesthesia is performed, puncture of the internal jugular vein and placement of the guide wire. Small skin incision at the place of exit of the guide wire (Fig. 2). Insertion of the dilator together with the peel-away tube in the internal jugular vein, removal of the dilator and insertion of the internal part of the catheter in the vein. Removal of the tube by peeling away. Correct placement of the catheter tip at the point of the entrance of the right atrium (controlled by radioscopy). Marking of the position of the dacron cuff on the skin (the subcutaneous loop of

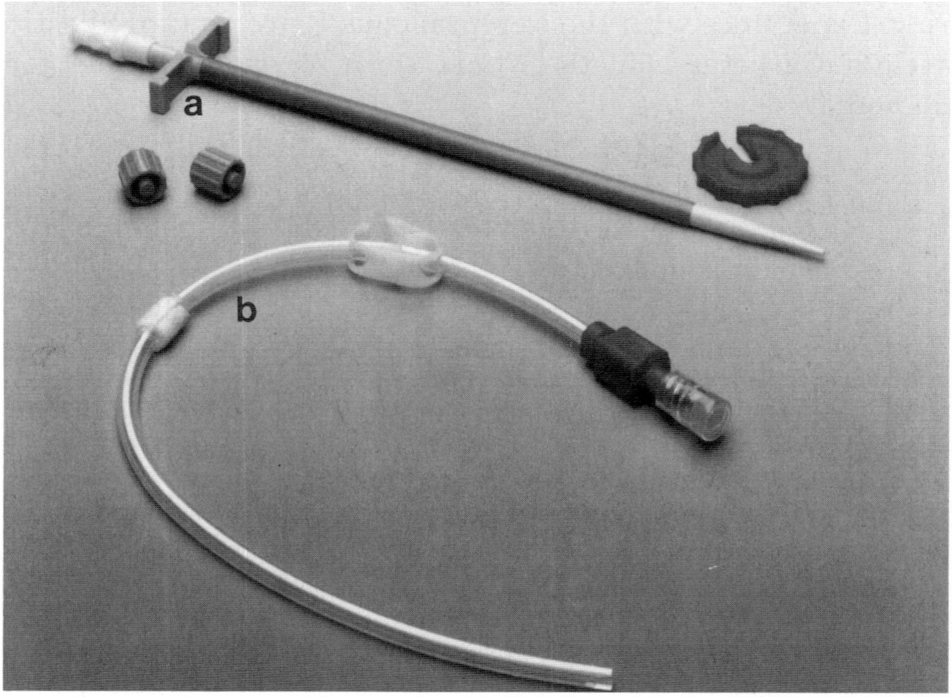

Fig. 1. (a) Dilator and 16 french peel-away tube. (b) Silastic catheter with dacron cuff and fish mouth shaped tip.

the catheter must be formed in a way, that this point is always placed caudal to the clavicula) and second skin incision just caudal to this marking. Placement of the external part of the catheter likewise with dilator and peel-away tube (Fig. 3). Stiches of the skin of both incisions (Fig. 4).

We used an implantable Silastic catheter (Bionic, Friedrichsdorf, FRG) with the following data: length 40 cm, outer diameter 4.8 mm, inner diameter 3 mm. A non on center dacron-cuff (1 cm long) divides the catheter into two different parts of 17 and 22 cm (type right) resp. 9 and 30 cm (type left). For different bodily sizes resp. sides of implantation (right/left) thereby 3 different internal parts (17, 22 and 30 cm) are available. The tip of the catheter is fish mouthed shaped to prevent suction at the vein wall. The catheter has no lateral holes.

Results

In the last 14 months we implanted 43 catheters as discribed. In three cases the puncture of the internal jugular vein was impossible. Two of these cases were successfully punctured with the aid of ultra sonic examination. The third patient had a thrombosed internal jugular vein (without punctures before).

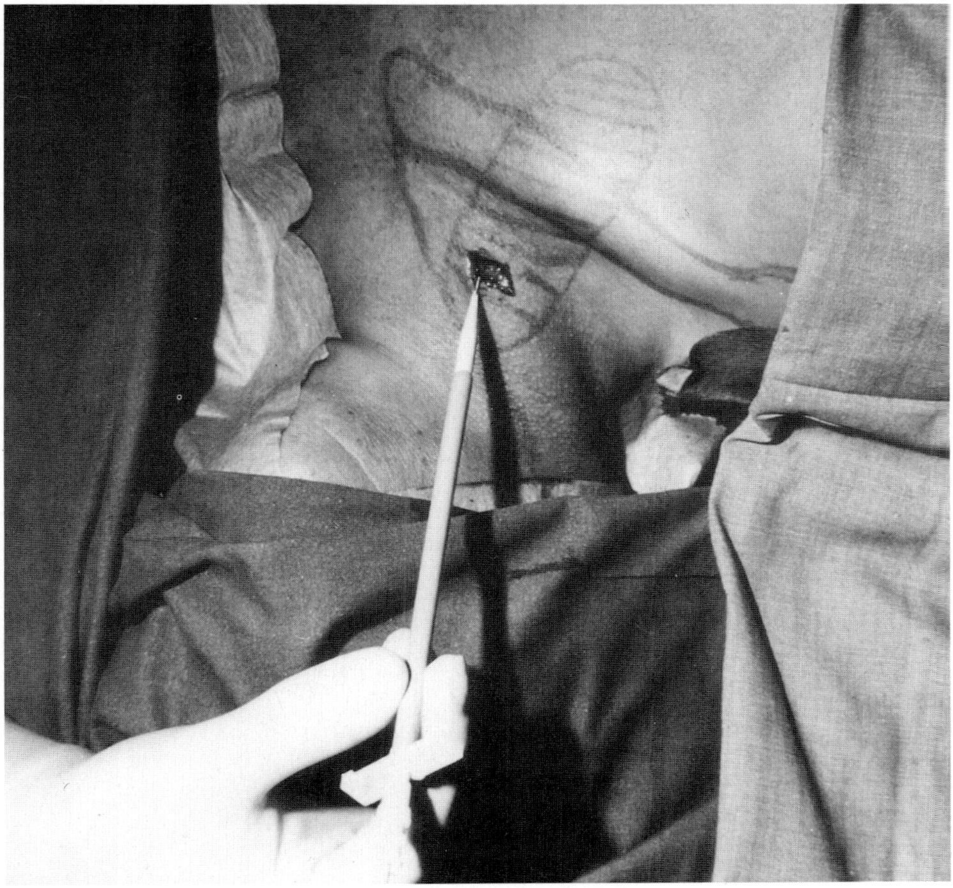

Fig. 2. Area of local anesthesia (shaded), guide wire in place, cranial skin incision, dilator and peel-away tube before insertion.

There were no complications in performing this puncture technique: no bleeding, no pneumothorax and no infection.

Discussion

The first vascular access devices for experimental and human dialysis were glass or plastic catheters placed by vasotomy. It was the merit of Shaldon to introduce the Seldinger-technique for the transcutaneous catheter placement by puncture, first arterio-venous, later on veno-venous because of high incidence of complications.

These catheters must be stiff and are formed like a dilator so that they can be punched over the guide wire into the vein. That is why the opening at the tip is

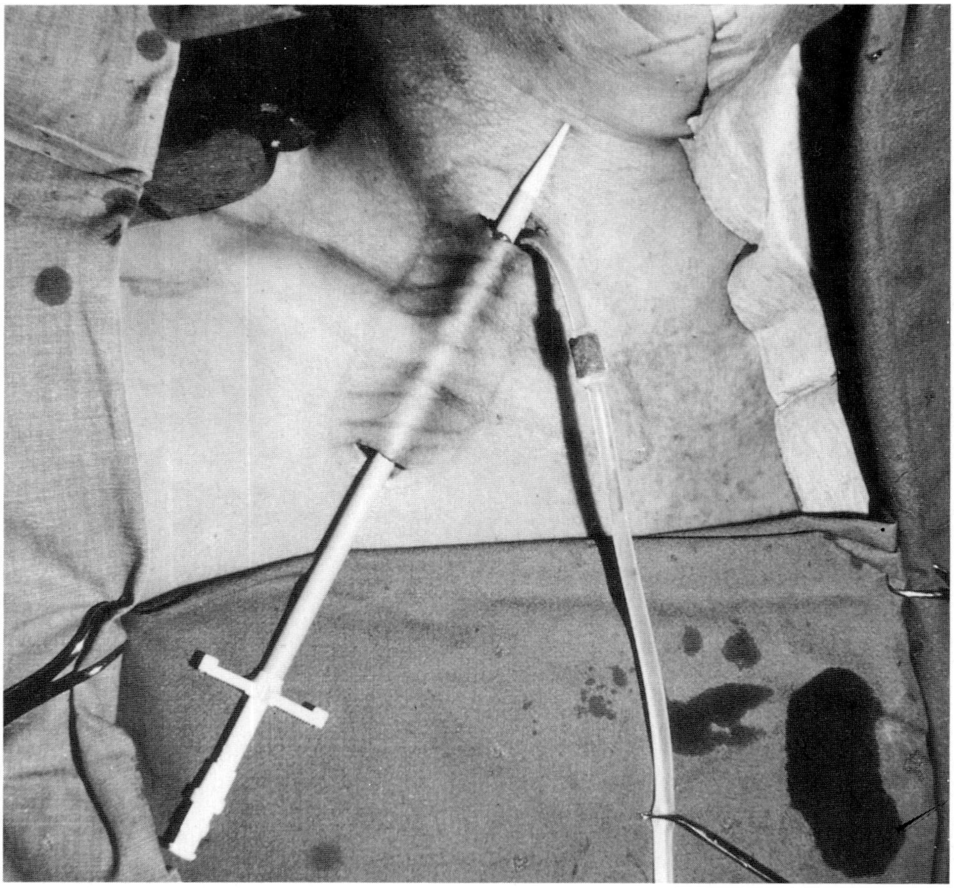

Fig. 3. Internal part of the catheter in place. Dilator and peel-away tube for the placement of the external part of the catheter in place.

very small. To obtain sufficient blood flow and to avoid suction of the vein wall these catheters need lateral holes. So often thrombosis occured in the segment with the lateral holes, because the infused heparin solution was washed out in a short time. The stiff catheters traumatized the vessel walls and were of much discomfort for the patients especially when placed into the internal jugular vein. Because of the induced stenoses and thromboses of the subclavian vein by puncture, this vein should not be used any longer for catheter placement.

These are some reasons why the smooth catheters without lateral holes and fish mouth shaped tip have a lot of advantages especially when placed in the internal jugular vein. The only disadvantage was the necessity to place the catheter by an operation. Since about two years a peel-away introducer set is available, which allows to place the smooth catheter by Seldinger-technique. We used this set in

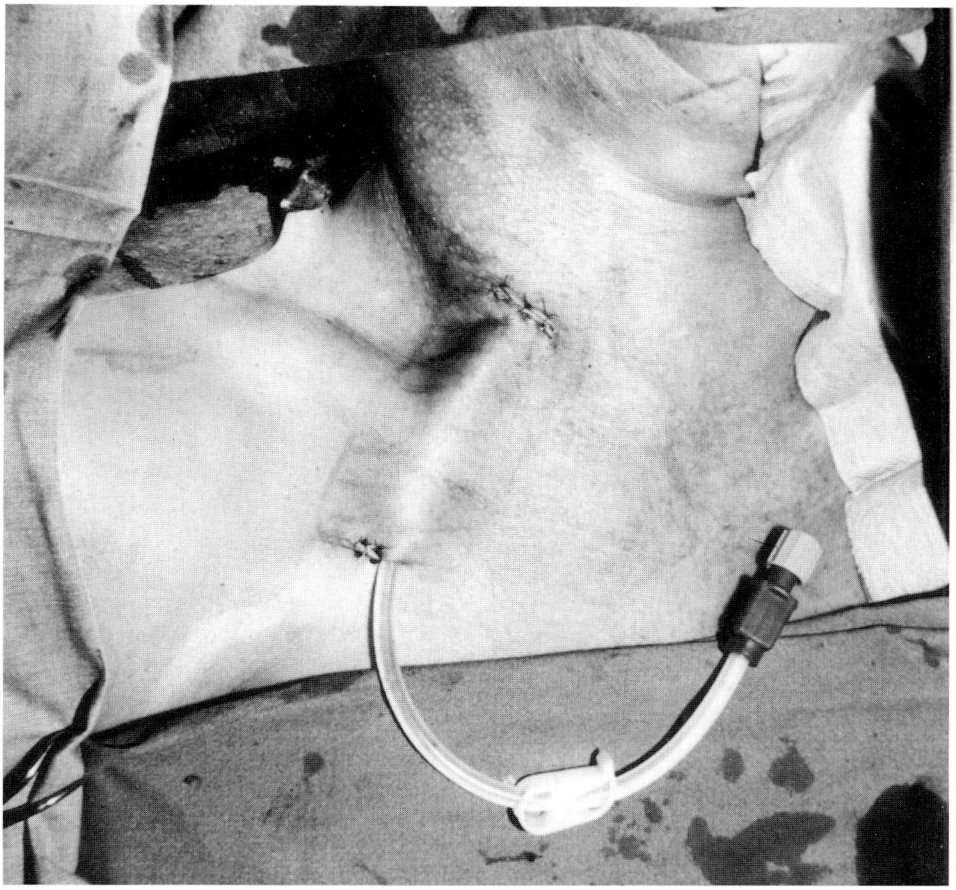

Fig. 4. Situs when the catheter placement is finished.

the last 14 months in 43 patients. The technique and results are described. The described method is fast and simple to perform with local anesthesia and can be done by the nephrologist. Although placed in the internal jugular vein the smooth catheter can be placed in a subcutaneous loop so that it steps out of the skin caudal of the clavicula. This means minimal discomfort for the patient.

With the development of the described technique we don't see an indication for the placement of catheters by operation in the internal jugular vein further on with the exception of those cases, when puncture technique despite an open internal jugular vein provoced by ultra sonic examination is not successful.

Comparison between Vascular Access for Immediate Hemodialysis

M. MOROSETTI, C. MELONI, L. MESCHINI, M. TACCONE-GALLUCCI, S. DI GIULIO, C. CASCIANI

Abstract

Different kinds of blood access devices have been used for immediate extracorporeal treatment: large catheters in deep veins as subclavian, internal jugular or femoral and external artero-venous shunts. The cannulation of deep veins can lead to severe complications such as stenosis or thrombosis of the vein, cervical hematomas, hemothorax, cardiac tamponade, or clotting of the catheter. An external artero-venous shunt is free from serious complications; moreover, according to our experience, it can be further converted into subcutaneous artero-venous fistula for patients in end stage renal failure. 96 patients needing immediate hemodialysis were operated and given vascular access in our department.

41 patients were treated by hemodialysis with large bore catheters in femoral or subclavian vein and 55 patients received an external artero-venous shunt.

In conclusion our data show that when immediate hemodialysis treatment is needed in end stage renal failure, the external artero-venous shunt is a better alternative to an intravenous catheter; moreover, the site of artero-venous shunt can further be used, after conversion into an artero-venous fistula, with higher blood flow, once the vein has been dilated with the external shunt.

Introduction

An internal artero-venous (AV) fistula is a first choice vascular access for hemodialysis treatment in end stage renal failure (ESRF) [1]. However an AV fistula cannot be used for regular puncture for days or weeks after surgery. In these conditions AV fistula cannot be considered as a quick vascular access for immediate treatment for acute renal failure (ARF) or late diagnosed ESRF.

Several kinds of vascular access have been suggested for immediate extracorporeal blood purification: either deep vein cannulation using indwelling catheters, femoral [2], subclavian [3], jugular [4], or implantation of external AV shunt [5]. Recently conversion of an AV external shunt into an internal AV fistula has been suggested when long term hemodialysis treatment is expected [6].

The aim of this work is to compare, according to our experience, the use for immediate hemodialysis treatment of external AV shunt further converted into an

AV fistula, versus that of catheters in deep veins. Function, incidence and severity of complications, stability and technical aspects are considered.

Patients and Methods

Since January 1985 until April 1988, 96 patients (mean age 59.4 ± 19.3 years range 28-72) were treated with immediate hemodialysis in our unit: 41 for ARF (group I) and 55 for rapidly progressive ESRF (group II).

Group I: In 28 patients a subclavian catheter (20 were double lumen, eight were single lumen catheters) was inserted into right atrium; the other 13 patients were hospitalized patients treated with catheters inserted into the vena cava through the femoral vein. All were Teflon catheters. The catheters were inserted only by designated members of the dialytic staff. Aseptic technique was employed at the time of catheter insertion and whenever the catheter was manipulated (declotting, connection with dialysis tubing, change of the cannula). Catheters were used only for dialysis treatment. Single lumen catheters were used with blood flow in single pass only. Catheters were inserted into deep veins according to Seldinger's procedure and sutured in place without subcutaneous tunneling; proper location of subclavian catheters was verified by chest x-rays. The catheter was not removed after each dialysis session and it was filled with saline and heparin (2,500 IU).

Table 1. Causes of ESRD in 55 patients treated with immediate hemodialysis.

Chronic glomerulonephritis	11	20.0 %
Chronic pyelonephritis	7	12.7 %
Nephroangiosclerosis	10	18.1 %
Polycystic renal disease	4	7.2 %
Diabetic nephropathy	7	12.7 %
Myeloma	3	5.4 %
Lupus nephropathy	1	1.8 %
Amyloidosis	2	3.6 %
Panarteritis nodosa	1	1.8 %
Unknown causes	9	16.3 %

Group II: Table 1 shows the causes of ESRD of the 55 patients of group II. All these patients underwent insertion of an external AV shunt between the radial artery and the cephalic vein according to a modified Ramirez technique [7]. Prothrombin activity was maintained within 50 % of control value with oral anticoagulant (dicumarol). In 47 patients the AV shunt was further converted into internal AV fistula after 28.3±10.3 days (range 17-35). When the external AV shunt was converted into AV fistula, the radial artery and the cephalic vein have already been dilated and they were stretched 2-2.5 cm proximal to the site of insertion of the cannulation tips; end to end anastomosis was created with running suture of polypropylene 6-0 or Goretex 7-0. Two or three days after the conversion, vascular tips of the external shunt were pulled out in order to prevent infection of the wound. Results are expressed as mean ± SD.

Results

Group I: 492 hemodialysis sessions were performed in 41 patients using catheters; blood flow range, during the dialysis sessions, was 200-300 ml/min. Hemodialysis treatment lasted 35.2±11.6 days (range 5-42). Failure of the catheter (obstruction, infection, low blood flow) leading to its replacement occured after 14.7±7.2 days. No severe complication was observed such as hemothorax, pneumothorax or cardiac tamponade. The incidence of the other early or late complications related with catheters are shown in Table 2. Catheters were replaced 13 times because of infection and 18 times because of obstructive thrombi.

Table 2. Incidence of early and late complications using deep vein catheters for immediate hemodialysis (Group I).

Early complications (recovering after manual compression)		
– puncture of the femoral artery	2	15.3 %
– puncture of the subclavian artery	2	7.1 %
Late complications		
– infection (chills, fever, positive culture of the catheter	13	31.7 %
subclavian vein	4	14.2 %
femoral vein	9	69.2 %
– clotting and/or occlusion of the catheters	18	43.9 %
dual lumen	13	44.8 %
single lumen	5	41.6 %
– phlebotrombosis of deep veins	5	12.1 %
subclavian vein	2	7.1 %
femoral vein	3	23.0 %

Group II: 1566 hemodialysis sessions were performed in 55 ESRF patients with an external AV shunt. The blood flow rate was ≥ 300 ml/min. Mean interval before the external shunt was converted into AV fistula was 28.9 ± 8.1 days (range 17-35 days). No severe complication was recorded such as sepsis or bleeding was observed. Some late complication was recorded: three episodes of local infection treated with antibiotics, six cases of clotting of AV shunt (repared in five cases with a Fogarty thrombectomy and needing once its full replacement), three cases of gastrointestinal bleeding recovered when anticoagulant treatment was withdrawn. The external AV shunt was converted into fistula in 47 of 55 patients, five patients died for causes unrelated with vascular access, two patients recovered from renal failure receiving then only conservative treatment, one new AV fistula was created on the contralateral forearm for failure of the previous one. In 46 of the 47 AV fistulas

(97.8 %), 2.5 ± 1.2 days (range 2-5) after conversion, blood flow was adequate for efficient dialysis treatment. Mean follow up of these AV fistulas was 21.0 ± 11.0 months (range 4-39); 25 of them are still working now for regular dialysis treatment. Among the 47 operated patients five died for reason unrelated with the vascular access, six were addressed to other dialysis units when the AV fistula was still working (unfortunately no information on the follow up is available today), 28 of the remaining 36 (78 %) AV fistulas are still functioning, while eight (22 %) failed, leading to a new vascular access, after a mean time of 14.3 ± 8.7 months (range 3-31) because of thrombosis.

Discussion

Vascular access suitable for immediate hemodialysis treatment has to provide the following features: easy and quick implantability, low incidence of complications, adequate and stable blood flow for extracorporeal circulation, sparing vessels for further vascular access in patients continuing regular dialysis treatment. Shaldon [2], Erben [3], and Bambauer [4] suggested deep vein cannulation, respectively femoral, subclavian and jugular vein, with catheters for immediate hemodialysis. These procedures allow quick insertion by experienced medical staff, mobility of the patients when the subclavian or jugular catheters are used and economy of sites for vascular access. Moreover double lumen catheters [8] allow hemodialysis treatment using a single vessel and conventional blood pumps. Several complications [9, 10], however, have been listed when deep veins are cannulated with catheters: local hematoma after accidental arterial puncture, local infection, clotting of the catheters, phlebitis and/or thrombosis. Major complications have also been reported: septicemia, hemothorax, pneumothorax and cardiac tamponade. Table 3 summarizes the incidence of major complications according to the literature. The external AV shunt, as described in 1960 by Quinton and Scribner [5], with technical modifications later suggested by others [7], can provide high and stable blood flow, adequate for immediate hemodialysis treatment, no severe complication has been recently reported with this procedure, moreover the patient is not immobilized like with femoral catheters. However this procedure has some drawbacks: surgical setting is necessary, anticoagulant treatment may be dangerous, generally the artery and the vein use for external AV shunt are lost for further vascular access, thus wasting one of the limited number of sites. Conversion of the external shunt into AV fistula according to Graben's procedure [6], can actually spare one of these sites yet providing quick vascular access for immediate hemodialysis. Venous catheters showed, in the present study, to be adequate for blood purification in different clinical conditions (i.e. ARF) with low incidence of complications.

Main complications were: infection and obstruction of the catheters, leading to their replacement. However, conversion of external shunt into an AV fistula

Table 3. Complications related to subclavian catheters for hemodialysis according to literature.

		No of patients	No of cases	%
Sepsis				
Vanholder	[15]	147	9	6.1
Uldall	[14]	64	9	14.0
Vanherweghem	[9]	148	17	11.5
Present study		41	5	12.1
Phlebothrombosis				
Vanholder	[15]	19*	13	68.4
Uldall	[14]	64	1	1.5
Vanherweghem	[9]	148	5	3.4
Present study		41	5	12.1
Hemothorax, cardiac tamponnade (for subclavian catheters only)				
Uldall	[14]	12	1	8.3
Vanherweghem	[9]	31	4	12.9
Present study		28	0	0.0

* Systematic phlebography

provided effective and stable blood flow in patients with chronic renal failure suddenly starting renal replacement therapy with hemodialysis. The incidence, however low, of complications was mainly related to the anticoagulant treatment of the external shunt and it can be reduced further, according to our recent experience, substituting platelet antiaggregants for dicumarols, and reducing the time of use of the shunt prior to its conversion into fistula. Function, after long term observation, of AV fistulas after conversion from external shunt was comparable with that of conventional AV fistulas as reported in the literature [11, 12, 13].

In conclusion, according to our experience and to the literature, a catheter in deep veins fulfill the optimal conditions requested for treatment of acute renal failure unless complications and instability of function are prevented; however the external shunt, further converted into AV fistula for emergency hemodialysis in patients with ESRF, provides high blood flow with low incidence of complications yet sparing one site for vascular access.

References

[1] Brescia, M. J., J. E. Cimino, K. Appel, et al.: Chronic hemodialysis using venipuncture and a surgically created arterievenous fistula. *N. Engl. J. Med.* 275: 1089 (1966).

[2] Shaldon, S., H. Silva, J. Pomeroy, A. L. Rae, S. M. Rosen: Percutaneous femoral venous catheterization and reusable dialysers in the treatment of acute renal failure. *Trans. Am. Soc. Artif. Int. Organs* 10: 133 (1964).

[3] Erben, J., J. Kvasnicka, J. Basteeky, V. Vortel: Experience with routine use of subclavian vein cannulation in hemodialysis. *Proc. Eur. Dial. Transplant. Assoc.* 6: 59-64 (1969).

[4] BAMBAUER, R., G. A. JUTZLER: Transcutaneous insertion of the Shaldon catheter through the internal jugular vein as access for acute hemodialysis. *Dial. Transpl.* 11: 766 (1982).

[5] QUINTON, W. E., D. DILLARD, B. N. SCRIBNER: Cannulation of blood vessels for prolonged hemodialysis. *Trans. Am. Soc. Artif. Int. Organs* 6: 104 (1960).

[6] GRABEN, N., A. DAUL, R. WINDECK: Successful conversion of external shunts to arterio-venous fistulas in adults and children with end-stage renal failure. *Trans. Am. Soc. Artif. Int. Organs* 29: 373 (1983).

[7] RAMIREZ, O., C. SWARTZ, G. ORESTE, et al.: The winged in line shunt. *Trans. Am. Soc. Artif. Int. Organs* 12: 220 (1966).

[8] RAJA, R. M., M. S. KRAMER, R. ALVIS, S. GOLDSTEIN, S. DELOSANGELES: A comparison of double lumen subclavian with single lumen catheters. One year experience. *Trans. Am. Soc. Artif. Int. Organs* 30: 508 (1984).

[9] VANHERWEGHEM, J. L., P. CABOLET, M. DHAENE, M. GOLDMAN, J. C. STOLEAR, J. P. SABOT, Y. WATERLOT, M. MARCHAL: Complications relate to subclavian catheters for hemodialysis. *Am. J. Nephrol.* 6: 339 (1986).

[10] ANDERSEN, J. T., J. GAMMELGAARD, L. M. NIELSEN, E. CLAUSEN: Subclavian vein catheterization for acute and chronic haemodialysis. A safe temporary vascular access. *Intern. Urol. Nephrol.* 18: 327-332 (1986).

[11] GEUN-EUN, K., H. HOVAGUIMIAN, R. MATALON: Vascular access for patients on long-term hemodialysis maintenance. *N. Y. State J. Med.* 84: 178 (1984).

[12] RIBET, M., J. P. CHAMBRON, G. DUVAL: Les fistulas arterio-veineuses pour hemodialise chronique. A propos de 400 cases. *Jour. Chir.* 119: 429 (1982).

[13] BALDRATI, L., P. PAGANELLI, G. ROMANELLI, et al.: La nostra esperienza sulle fistole artero-venose interne come accesso vascolare per l'emodialisi. *Minerva Chirurgica* 42: 385 (1987).

[14] ULDALL, P. R., R. F. DIJCK, F. WOODS, N. MERCHANT, G. S. MARTIN, C. J. CARDELLA, D. M. C. SUTTON, G. A. DE VEBER: A subclavian catheter for temporary vascular access for hemodialysis or plasmapheresis. *Dial. Transpl.* 8: 963 (1979).

[15] VANHOLDER, R., N. LAMEIRE, J. VERBANCK, R. VAN RATTINGHE, M. KAMNEN, S. RINGOIR: Complications of subclavian catheters hemodialysis: a 5-years prospective study in 257 consecutive patients. *Int. J. Artif. Organs* 5: 297 (1982).

A Modified Right Atrial Silicone Catheter for Access to Circulation for Chronic Hemodialysis Treatment

M. Malovrh, J. Drinovec, R. Ponikvar, A. Guček, J. Varl

Abstract

Since March 1986 until October 1988, 11 Francis silicone catheters placed in the right atrium were used as long-term vascular access to circulation for chronic hemodialysis. The patients were retrospectively evaluated for catheter usefulness and catheter related complications. The cumulative usefulness of 18 months was 54 %. In three cases there were exit site infections with sepsis, in three cases catheter thrombosis and three patients had local hematoma in the neck after insertion of the catheter. Two patients died for other reasons with patent catheters. At the end of the study, four catheters are still functioning.

Introduction

Vascular access has always been the most important and the most limiting factor in the success of hemodialysis [1, 2]. In some patients with poor vessels and hypotension, arteriovenous fistulas (AVF) are useful for a short time [1]. When all conventional sides have been exhausted the right atrium single lumen silicone catheter as long-term vascular access for chronic hemodialysis (HD) can be used [1, 2].

Patients and Methods

From March 1986 to October 1988, 11 Francis catheters were used in nine patients treated with chronic HD. There were six women and three men, ages from 38 to 79 years, mean 59 ± 13 years. They were treated with chronic HD from 12 to 120 months, mean 54 ± 40 months. The number of previous vascular accesses was from three to seven.

We used Francis silicone single lumen catheters with two Dacron cuffs (Quinton, USA). The catheter length was 42 cm, internal diameter 3.0 mm, external diameter 5.0 mm, the length of cuff was 1 cm. Insertion of the catheter was done by a vascular surgeon, using the cut-down method in sterile conditions and under fluoroscopy control. The tip of the catheter was placed at the junction of the superior vena cava and right atrium. The other side was advanced through the subcutaneous tunnel to the exit site 1-2 cm under the nipple. Nine catheters were inserted through the right internal jugular vein and two through the left. When the catheters were not in use, they had been flushed with 2.5 ml of heparin.

Results

Characteristics of patients with Francis catheters, time of the catheter usefulness and reasons for their removal are shown on Table 1. Three catheters were thrombosed, two of them were inserted through the left internal jugular vein. In three patients there were exit site infections with sepsis, and two catheters had to be removed. In one of these patients, because of dense subcutaneous adhesions of the Dacron cuffs only a part of the catheter was removed. Three patients had local hematoma in the neck after insertion. Two patients died for other reasons with patent catheter. At the end of our study, four catheters were still functioning.

Table 1. Characteristics of patients with Francis catheters, time of catheter usefulness and reason for his removal (n = 11).

Patient	Age (years)	Number of vascular accesses	Time of usefulness (days)	Reason for removal
1	62	3	113	thrombosis
2	62	3	42	death
3	38	4	1	thrombosis
4	53	7	9	thrombosis
5	50	6	598	sepsis, new fistula
6	38	6	883	–
7	52	4	149	sepsis, new fistula
8	79	2	400	–
9	61	3	55	death
10	79	3	137	–
11	56	2	130	–

Conclusions

A Francis right atrium single lumen silicone catheter as long-term vascular access for chronic HD is useful, especially for those patients with poor vessels and hypotension. For most of them this catheter as a long-term vascular access is the last chance. The Francis catheter must always be inserted through the right internal jugular vein. Complications are not rare but with careful handling the catheter may be kept in function for a long time.

References

[1] Butt, K. M. H.: Angioaccess, pp. 171-85. In: Drukker, W., F. M. Person, J. F. Maher (eds.): Replacement of renal function by dialysis. Martinus Nijhoff Publ.: Boston 1983.

[2] Stabile, B. E.: Vascular access for total parenteral nutrition, pp. 5-51. In: Wilson, S. E., M. L. Owens (eds.): Vascular access surgery. Year Book Medical Publ.: Chicago 1980.

Fibrin Sheet Covering Subclavian or Femoral Dialysis Catheters

R. Hombrouckx, F. D'Halluin, A. M. Bogaert, F. Leroy,
J. Y. De Vos, L. Larno

Abstract

The suspicion of the existence of a sheet around the single lumen dialysis catheter-tip, provoking a valve mechanism, is from the observation that several times during the replacement procedures of a dialysis catheter, a sheet, surrounding the surface of the catheter, is removed together with the dialysis catheter. This sheet is grey ca. 1 mm thick and ca. 30 mm long and bacteriological examinations are always negative.

The existence of the sheet in vivo is demonstrated by digitalized angiography during the removing procedure of the single lumen dialysis catheter. In exceptions only the sheet is removed together with the catheter. In all other instances the sheet is stripped off and remains in the subcutaneous tunnel or in the vascular bed, obviously without causing much clinical discomfort in most cases.

Occasionally an episode of cough, dyspnoe, hypotension, retrosternal oppression or hemoptoe, after removing the single lumen dialysis catheter, suggests pulmonary embolization or lung infarction.

Introduction

It often happens that a single lumen dialysis catheter (SLDC) in combination with a single needle dialysis system, allows a good venous return, but not a good arterial supply, suggesting a sort of valve mechanism in, or around the SLDC-tip.

Materials

The routine SLDC we used were:
- Extracorporeal FC 100, made of Teflon
- Gambro Vas-Cath SC 2100, made of polyurethane
- Miramed Uni-Cath 370, made of polyurethane
- Medcomp 01CMD240, made of polyurethane

Methods

The SLDC are routinely treated in the following way after each dialysis session:
- rinse with about 10 ml of saline,
- filling up with about 1.5 ml of heparin (= catheter content),
- lock up with a Luer-Lock cap.

Whenever there is a problem of bad arterial supply, kinking, thrombosis a.s.o., the catheter is replaced by a routine Seldinger replacement technique. Even in the absence of any clinical problem, the SLDC is replaced every five weeks in order to prevent mechanical disjunction. The definitive SLDC removal was during two years routinely done under digitalized angiography.

Results

The suspicion of the existence of a sheet around the SLDC-tip, provoking a valve mechanism, is from the observation that several times, during replacement procedures of a SLDC, a sheet, surrounding the surface of the SLDC is removed together with the SLDC.

This sheet is grey, about 1 mm thick and about 30 mm long and consists of fibrin and thrombocytes.

Bacteriological examinations are always negative.

The existence of the sheet in vivo is demonstrated by a digitalized angiography during the removing procedure of the SLDC.

Discussion and Conclusion

Only exceptionally the sheet is removed together with the SLDC, in all other instances the sheet is stripped off and remains in the subcutaneous tunnel or in the vascular bed, obviously without causing much clinical discomfort in most cases.

Occasionally, an episode of cough, dyspnoe, hypotension, retrosternal oppression or hemoptysis, after the removing of a SLDC, suggests pulmonary embolization or lung infarction symptoms.

A New 2-Compartment-Catheter for Systematic Drainage from Hepatic Veins to Extracorporeal Space. First Results in Animal Studies

M. V. HELZEL

Abstract

A new therapeutic catheter – the 2-compartment-catheter – for systematic drainage from hepatic veins to extracorporal space without blocking of caval blood flow to right atrium is presented.

Its principle is outlined. First results in animal trial are referred.

With two additional catheters isolated liver perfusion in exclusive catheter technique without laparotomy becomes possible for various therapeutic intentions: in oncology, traumatology, pharmacology, intensive care in intoxications with acute liver failure and chronic phacomatoses of the liver.

Introduction

The first experiences in animal studies with a new therapeutic catheter are reported. This 2-compartment-catheter permits separate drainage of blood from hepatic veins to extracorporal space – without affecting caval blood flow. With additional use of two commercially available angiographic catheters, isolated liver-perfusion in this exclusive catheter technique becomes possible.

On the pre-hepatic side catheterization of the hepatic artery or percutaneous transhepatic puncture of the portal vein are established methods. On the post-hepatic side the separate drainage from hepatic veins was not possible until recently.

Main difficulties exist in separating blood volume of hepatic veins (compartment 1) and blood volume of vena cava (compartment 2):

- There is a high volume of flow up to 40 to 50 ml/sec in the inferior vena cava in humans.
- Junctions of hepatic veins to vena cava inferior are irregular in the distance between the diaphragm and renal veins.

Complete drainage of mixed blood from both compartments for extracorporal dialysis is possible and is proposed by Aigner [1, 2].

The disadvantage of Aigner's method is its expenditure (laparotomy) and the possible hemolysis because of high blood volume for hemofiltration of oncologic drugs.

Principle of 2-compartment-catheter

The 2-compartment-catheter (US patent No 915.050, German patent No 35 35 641.3) consists of a 3-luminal trunk: two lumina serve for balloon-expansion, another lumen for drainage from blood of hepatic veins. There is an additional (fourth) lumen at the top of the catheter: a large calibrated cylinder with two ring-balloons in a certain distance. A great central opening permits passage of caval blood back to the right atrium.

The insertion of this catheter requires open femoral venotomy because of its configuration and size at the top.

Materials and Methods

35 studies in 35 animals (16-22 Kg dogs) were performed. Trials with ruptured ring-balloons (n =4) were not evaluated. The 2-compartment-catheter, introduced transfemorally by open venotomy, was placed in the inferior vena cava with its cranial ring-balloon at a height of the right diaphragm (under fluoroscopic guidance). After that, three different modes of contrast medium applications were performed:

1. Via truncus coeliacus, by sondation with a diagnostic catheter type Sidewinder I, (n=11).
2. Via portal vein, by percutaneous transhepatic puncture (n=6).
3. Via contralateral iliac vein, by percutaneous puncture (n=14).

After extension of the two ring-balloons of the 2-compartment-catheter iodine contrast medium (1 ml Ultravist / kg body weight) was injected by one of the above mentioned application-modes.

The purpose of these trial-arrangements was, to prove differences in concentrations of contrast medium between the two compartments: region of junctions of hepatic veins (compartment 1) and vena cava inferior (compartment 2).

Determination of iodine concentrations in the two compartments was performed by fluorescense-photometry [3, 4]: measurements by double values in homogenous 10 % KOH-solution.

Results

Depending on the mode of contrast medium application, different concentrations of iodine were observed in simultaneously taken blood samples in the two compartments (12-18 blood probes in intervals of three seconds were per-

Table 1. Iodine concentration.

Current number	Vena cava inferior	Regions of liver veins inflow
1	0.135	0.194
2	0.137	0.700
3	0.139	3.874
4	0.138	11.034
5	0.139	15.448
6	0.133	16.297
7	0.134	11.436
8	0.157	8.099
9	0.313	6.274
10	0.478	5.187
11	0.754	4.359
12	0.924	3.721
13	1.343	3.066
14	0.958	3.721
15	0.906	2.968
16	0.734	2.775
17	1.470	2.944
18	1.103	2.966

Contrast medium concentration (mg Iodine / g blood) in simultaneous taken blood samples of vena cava (compartment 2) and region of inflow from hepatic veins (compartment 1). Contrast bolus (1 ml Ultravist / kg body weight) via portal vein. Fluorescense-photometric measurement with double values in homogenous 10%-KOH solution. Current numbers indicate equal intervals of taken blood probes (3 sec). Sample size n = 6.

formed). Characteristic time-iodine-concentration relationships were obtained (Table 1, 2).

The average concentrations are reported:

After contrast medium application via truncus coeliacus differences of iodine concentration in the two compartments were 10-11 fold higher in compartment 1 than in the compartment 2.

Contrast medium application via portal vein showed high differences of iodine concentration in the two compartments in the range between 100-120 fold (Table 1).

Table 2 (contrast medium is applicated via iliac vein) shows maximum differences in iodine concentration between two compartments – factor 1,000-10,000. Because of the mode of contrast medium application, an inverse gradient in the two compartments is received.

The lower differences in iodine concentration in the two compartments after pre-hepatic application modes are explained by dilution of contrast medium by additional blood volume of portal vein respectively coeliac axis.

Additional reasons are:

a) leakage between surface of ring balloons and wall of vena cava;

b) the distance between the two ring-balloons could not be adapted to each animal, because of limited numbers of catheter prototypes: additional inflow of renal blood was possible and reduced differences in iodine concentrations between the two compartments.

Table 2. Iodine concentration.

Current number	Vena cava inferior	Regions of liver veins inflow
1	22.215	> 0.005
2	27.126	0.068
3	34.247	0.009
4	20.987	0.083
5	15.144	0.069
6	11.788	0.034
7	12.034	0.034
8	10.851	> 0.005
9	9.350	> 0.005
10	10.106	> 0.005
11	9.202	> 0.005
12	5.726	> 0.005

Same parameters and determination method respectively trial arrangement like in Table 1. Application of contrast medium via iliac vein. Sample size n = 14.

Discussion

Results in animal trials show that systematic separation of inflow from the hepatic veins (compartment 1) and blood volume of vena cava inferior (compartment 2) becomes possible; the 2-compartment-catheter permits this separation via open femoral venotomy without laparotomy and without total blocking of caval blood flow: the passage of caval blood to right atrium is maintained all along.

A target-conflict in isolated drainage from hepatic veins is caused by the two different functions of the 2-compartment-catheter: on the one hand not completely avoidable alteration of caval blood back-flow should be minimized; therefore catheter cross-section at its top should approximate the diameter of vena cava (3-4 cm in humans); on the other hand the size of the catheter-head should be small for easy introduction of the catheter via the peripheral venous system.

The observed iodine concentration differences between the two compartments can be used for therapeutic intentions: with additional use of two commercial angiographic-catheters, isolated liver perfusion in the exclusive catheter technique becomes practicable. The use of 2-compartment-catheter in humans could be:

1. Oncologic application: Isolated liver perfusion for short-termed high dose chemotherapy in primary or secondary liver neoplasms. Hemodialysis of blood from hepatic veins for elimination of cytotoxic drugs avoids systemic side effects.

2. Intensive care application: Isolated liver perfusion in acute liver-dystrophy (i.e. caused by acute intoxication, acute phase of cirrhosis) combined with detoxication either by pig liver perfusion or by hemodialysis [5].
3. Application in metabolic diseases: Application of 2-compartment-catheter for drug perfusion in phacomatoses i.e. chelats in hemochromatosis or Morbus Wilson and in phacomatoses in childhood.
4. Application in traumatology: Use of 2-compartment-catheter in polytrauma with central rupture of liver; esp. in tear-out of liver veins.
5. Pharmacological studies of metabolism of drugs in hepatocyts.

References

[1] AIGNER, K. R., H. J. HELLING, K. H. LINK, H. WALTHER, G. BILL, : Zytostatikafiltration unter regionaler Chemotherapie. *Beitr. Onkol.* 21: 229-245 (1985).

[2] AIGNER, K. R., J. C. TONN, R. HECHTEL, R. SEUFFER: Die intra-arterielle Zytostatikatherapie mit venöser Filtration im halboffenen System. *Onkologie* 6: 74-76 (1983).

[3] BELL, G. D., J. MCCULLIN, J. OLIVER, J. MCALISTER: A simple spectrophotometric method for measuring biliary ioglamide (Biligram) concentration. *Brit. J. Radiol.* 51: 17-19 (1978).

[4] EDHOLM, P., B. JACOBSON: Quantitative determination of iodine in vivo. *Acta Radiol.* 52: 337-346 (1959).

[5] SILK, D. B., N. TREWBY, R. A. CHASE, P. G. MELLON, M. A. HANID, M. DAVIES: Treatment of fulminant hepatic failure by polyacrylonitrilmembrane haemodialysis. *Lancet* II: 1-3 (1977).

Transluminal Angioplasty in the Treatment of Stenotic Dialysis Vascular Access: An Evaluation

E. MANGEL, H. SCHIFFL, K. J. PFEIFER

Abstract

The impaired function of hemodialysis shunts by stenoses or occlusions often and especially in multimorbid patients poses severe problems for therapeutic consequences. The aim of the present study was to determine the criteria for and effectiveness of angioplasty.

Within one year, percutaneous transluminal angioplasty of stenotic hemodialysis fistulas was performed in 12 patients. Traumatization and bleeding danger was markedly reduced by the use of 5F dilatation-catheters. Therefore, the procedure could be done under outpatient conditions.

The success rate is best in single or multiple short stenoses in both, Cimino shunts and synthetic grafts. The overall success rate of percutaneous transluminal angioplasty in our patients was 82 %, with a patency rate of 66 % at six months and of 63 % at 12 months, which is well comparable with the results of surgery.

The results of this study suggest: angioplasty can be done on an outpatient basis; it can be repeated several times; there is no risk from surgery or anesthesia; costs are considerably reduced.

Introduction

Satisfactory vascular access is an essential requirement for maintenance hemodialysis. The preferred access site is the internal arteriovenous fistula. When an artery and an adequate vein are not in close proximity, prosthetic conduits may be constituted.

Access to the circulation remains, however, the Achilles heel of these patients. Failure of dialysis fistulas is commonly due to the occurrence of stenoses in the venous or, less frequently, the arterial limb. The resultant low blood flow causes inefficient dialysis and less optimal control of uremia, electrolyte and fluid imbalance.

Surgical repair of such stenotic lesions is often complex for the surgeon, threatening to the patient and may result in the loss of a given vascular access. Sporadic reports have appeared of successful dilation of stenotic lesions in dialysis fistulas. Our approach to the failing vascular access and the experience obtained

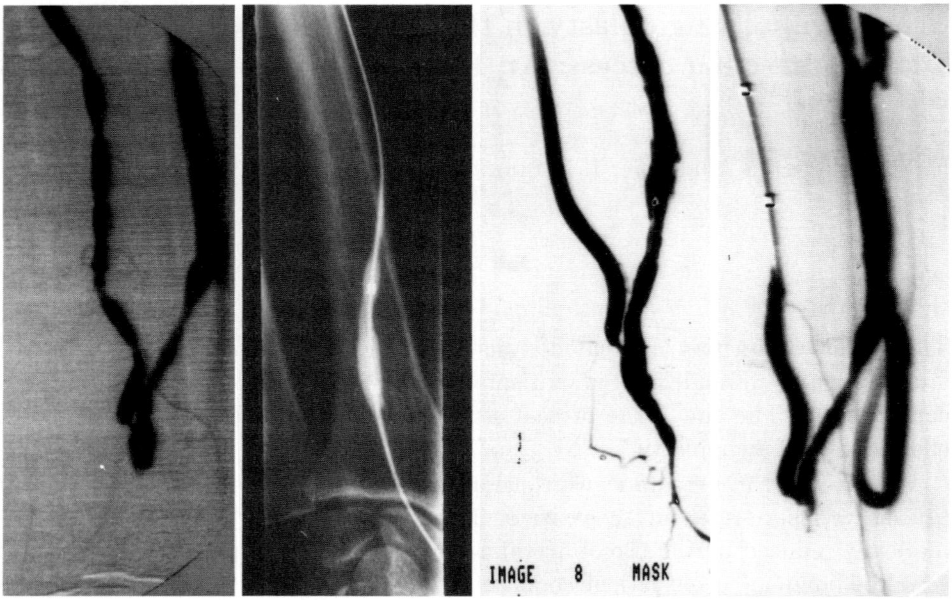

Fig. 1. a) AV-Fistula: Stenoses in the venous limb (arrow) and the access site. b) PTA of the venous limb. Bulging of the balloon. c) DSA after PTA of the venous limb. d) DSA after PTA of the access site.

with percutaneous transluminal angioplasty (PTA) in unselected consecutive cases form the basis of this report.

Patients and Methods

Seventeen stenotic lesions in the vascular access of 12 hemodialysis patients (six women, six men, mean age 67 years, range 50-82 years) were treated by PTA. Three percutaneous angioplasty procedures were performed in one patient, and two procedures were done in each of three patients. The cause of chronic renal failure was diabetic nephropathy in eight patients, chronic glomerulonephritis or chronic interstitial nephritis in two patients each. The vascular access was an internal arteriovenous fistula, an autologous graft and a prosthetic graft in four patients each.

The patients were referred for angiographic studies after documentation of access malfunction (decreased or absent blood flow or venous hypertension) during hemodialysis. Doppler ultrasonography, Duplex scan and angiogram of the vascular access were obtained according to standard techniques. The interpretation of the radiologic findings were reviewed with the nephrologist, the vascular surgeon and the radiologist, and a joint decision was made to attempt PTA. The majority of the stenoses were located at the venous limb, but some stenotic lesions were found at the anastomosis site or even at the arterial limb. The preferred access for PTA was through the distal or proximal vein. Heparin (5000 units given intravenously) was administered after the stenotic lesion was crossed with a straight guide wire.

Angioplasty balloons of 4 to 10 mm in diameter were used for dilatation and up to three inflations one minute each were employed. High pressure balloons (12 atmospheres) were used for anastomotic lesions. After the PTA an angiography was obtained in each case. All the diagnostic and therapeutic procedures were carried out in the outpatient department.

Results

All patients were followed up. Success was defined as patency of the vascular access for at least six months, patency of even less than six months at the time of this report, or patency until the patient's death. PTA was successful in 13 of 17 attempts (82 %). The six months patency rate was 66 %. One patient died within 12 months after PTA with a functioning graft. Two angioaccesses failed within 12 months after PTA. The success rate of 12 months or longer was 63 % on the basis of the above criteria. Typical examples documents the sequence of the procedure in various types of dialysis access are shown in Figures 1-3.

Primary failures of PTA occured in four cases. Two technical failures were in lesions that were originally considered poor candidates for PTA: a kinking of the venous limb and a high-grade anastomotic lesion. These lesions could not be negotiated with the guide wire. The patients required surgical revision. The two other failures were due an immediate thrombosis in a high-grade and tortuous venous segment and due to restenosis and thromboses at one week after PTA. In both patients surgical revision was successfully performed. Other complications were extremely low and consisted of one self-limited hematoma.

Discussion

Angioaccess is the most important determinant for the continuous well being of patients with end stage renal disease who are supported on hemodialysis. The most common problem with both internal arteriovenous fistulas or grafts is venous stenoses at or near the anastomotic site and resultant thrombosis and loss of the angioaccess. Patients with systemic vasculopathies and or increasing age may now be enrolled in chronic programs and experience the incessant fear of loss their "life-line".

Our evaluation of PTA in such a patient population prone to recurrent fistula failure demonstrates that this procedure is an ideal method for accomplishing

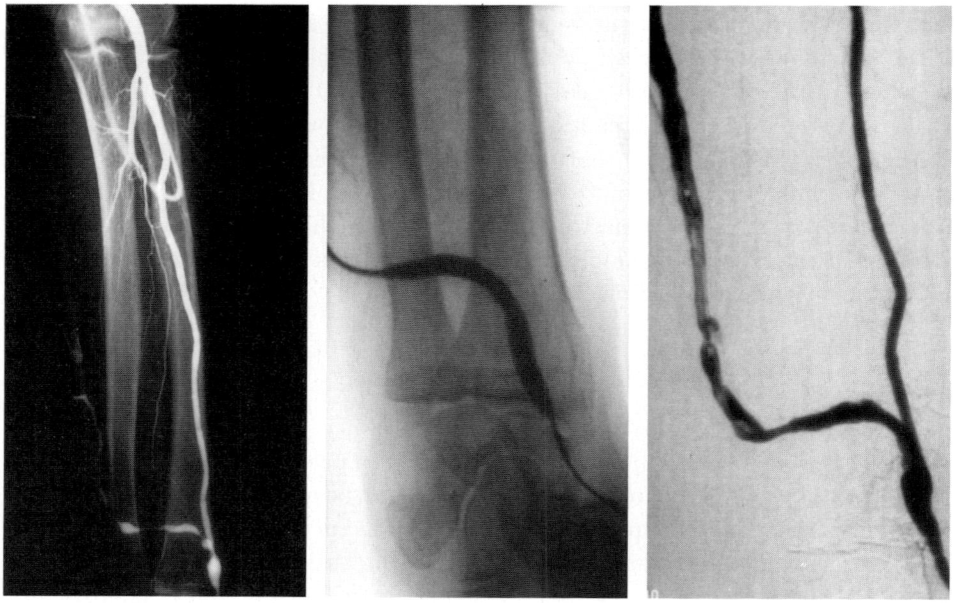

Fig. 2. a) Conventional shunt angiogram: Multiple stenoses in the autologous venous graft (arrows). b) PTA of the venous graft. c) Results of PTA of the graft.

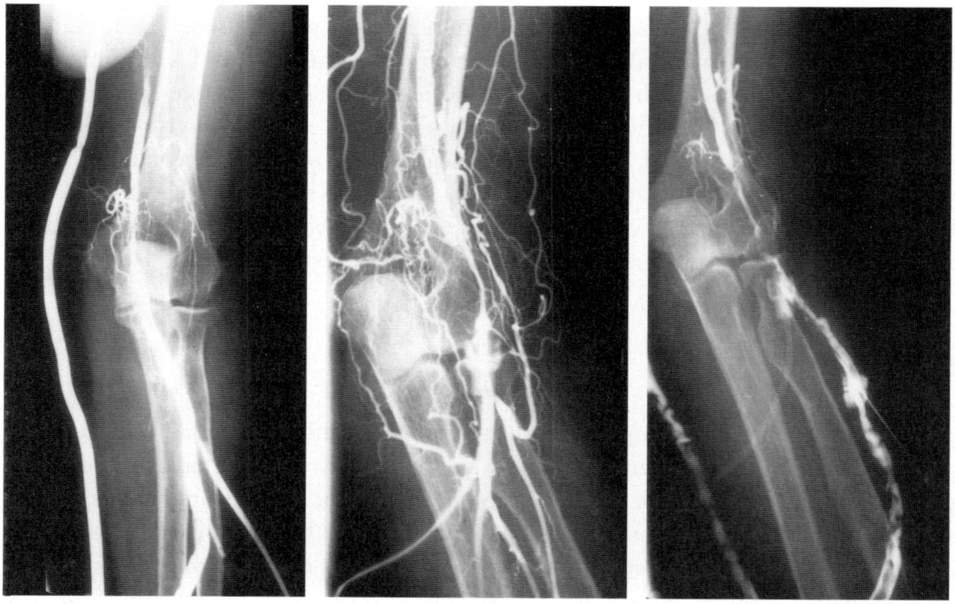

Fig. 3. a) Shunt angiogram: Stenosis of access site (brachial artery/Goretex graft). b) Angiogram one week after PTA: Occlusion of the loop. c) Thrombosis of the loop.

the preservation of vascular access for the maximal possible time. The overall success rate of PTA in our patients was 82 %, with a patency rate of 66 % at six months and of 63 % at 12 months. These cumulative patency rates after PTA are in accord with other studies [1-5] and may be almost twice as great as after surgical revision [1]. Even lower long-term patency rates from a single dilation may, however, be misleading since repeat angioplasty can easily be performed to prolong the life of angioaccess for years [2].

Whether or not the particular types of hemodialysis access may behave as distinct groups remains unclear. The success rate is best in single or multiple short stenoses for proximal anastomosis, but is not insignificant in more complicated cases. In contrast to other authors [2, 3] an attempt of PTA is justified even in cases with stenoses longer than 4 cm or prosthetic grafts. As any success saves a surgical intervention, this procedures should be done.

Primary failure were due to either to technical inability to pass the stenoses (two patients) or to thromboses during or shortly after the attempt. Compared to the surgical alternative of progressive depletion of access sites PTA is less threatening to patients than surgery, and the generally satisfactory results are associated with a low frequency of complications. Failure of a PTA attempt still allows surgical treatment. More importantly, after angioplasty the fistula can immediately be used for dialyses. PTA also reduces the need of subsequent invasive interventions such as implantation of temporary access device, and thus reduces the duration of hospitalizations.

In conclusion, percutaneous transluminal angioplasty is the treatment of choice for patients who have suitable lesions for the procedure. It can be performed on an outpatient basis immediately after diagnostic angiography. Intravascular stenting of venous outflow stenosis combined with PTA may probably prolong shunt patency and may be regarded as further benefit [6]. Surgery may be the preferred treatment for vascular access that fail before maturing adequately, since such early failure implies technical deficiencies in their construction, such as poor choice of vein, inadequate anastomosis, or unfavorable site of fistula placement. Long segment stenosis, particularly of prosthetic grafts, may have an unfavorable prospect of salvage by PTA and should like acute thrombosis of vascular access be treated by surgical intervention.

References

[1] Cada, E., F. Karnel, G. Mayer, F. Längle, H. Schurawitzki, H. Graf: Percutaneous transluminal angioplasty of failing arteriovenous fistulae. *Nephrol. Dial. Transplant.* 4: 57-61 (1989).

[2] Glanz, S., D. H. Gordon, K. M. Butt, J. Hong, R. Adamson, S. J. A. Sclafani: Stenotic lesions in dialysis-access fistulas: treatment by transluminal angioplasty using high-pressure balloons. *Radiology* 156: 236 (1985).

[3] GORDON, D. H., S. GLANZ, K. M. BUTT, R. ADAMSON, M. A. KOENIG: Treatment of stenotic lesions in dialysis access fistulas and shunts by transluminal angioplasty. *Radiology* 142: 53-58 (1982).

[4] RODRIGUEZ-PEREZ, J. C., M. MAYNAR, A. RAMS, C. PLAZA, N. VEGA, R. ALAMO, R. REYES, A. FERNANDEZ, L. PALOP: Percutaneous transluminal angioplasty as best treatment in stenosis of vascular access for hemodialysis. *Nephron* 51: 192-196 (1989).

[5] SAEED, M., G. E. NEWANN, R. L. MCCANN, S. K. SUSSMAN, S. D. BRAUN, N. R. DUNNICK: Stenoses of dialysis fistulas: treatment with percutaneous angioplasty. *Radiology* 164: 693-697 (1987).

[6] GÜNTHER, R. W., D. VORWERK, K. BOHNDORF, K. C. KLOSE, D. KISTLER, H. MANN, H. G. SIEBERTH, A. EL-DIN: Venous stenoses in dialysis shunts: treatment with self-expanding metallic stents. *Radiology* 170: 401-405 (1989).

Self-Expanding Metallic Stent for the Treatment of Dialysis Shunt Stenoses

D. VORWERK, R. W. GÜNTHER, K. BOHNDORF, D. KISTLER, H. MANN, H. G. SIEBERTH

Abstract

Self-expandable stents were implanted in nine failing hemodialysis fistulae. In all cases, balloon angioplasty alone yielded an unsatisfactory result, but flow could be successfully reestablished by stent placement in eight of nine cases. During a mean follow-up period of eight months restenosis occured in four of eight patients, but was successfully treated by percutaneous means. Stent placement seems to improve acute results following unsuccessful percutaneous treatment; long term results may be limited by recurrent stenosis due to intimal hyperplasia.

Introduction

Stenoses of hemodialysis fistulae often present therapeutic difficulties both in percutaneous balloon dilatation and operative revision. We wish to describe application of self-expandable vascular endoprostheses as an adjunct to balloon dilatation in nine cases of hemodialysis fistulae.

Materials and Methods

Nine patients (four women, five men) with venous stenoses of hemodialysis shunts were treated. At the time of treatment the shunt was totally thrombosed in six patients, in two patients the flow was markedly impaired due to severe stenoses. In one patient, the distal subclavian vein was totally occluded but venous flow was maintained by a network of collaterals. The shunt type was a PTFE shunt in five and an endogeneous shunt in four patients; all stenoses occurred in the venous part of the fistulae.

After balloon dilatation the stenotic areas were scaffolded by vascular endoprostheses varying between 3.5 and 16 cm in length and 7 to 8 mm in diameter. The implantation was controlled by fluoroscopy. In three patients stents did not fully expand after implantation and required additional balloon dilatation by suitable balloon catheters.

All procedures were performed under local anesthesia. During the procedure the patients received 5000 U of heparin. Postprocedural treatment included infusion of heparin (1000 U/h) and anti-platelet aggregation medication. Follow-up was performed clinically by DSA and color-coded duplex sonography.

Results

In all patients we were confronted with complicated problems, because all patients had undergone several shunt operations or revisions and potentials of new shunt anastomoses were low. All patients had undergone previous dilatation with insufficient results. In six patients thrombectomy had to be performed before stent implantation.

In eight patients the immediate result was successful. In one patient the shunt reoccluded within 12 hours after dilatation and was abandoned. In one patient the shunt occluded 12 hours after stent implantation, but could be thrombectomized one week later. Additional stent implantation was necessary in this case to restore shunt function. Residual stenosis in another patient also required early additional stent placement.

Follow-up time lasted from 1 to 14 months (mean 8.1 months). Shunt thrombosis occurred in one patient two months after implantation due to nocturnal hypotension, but thrombectomy was successful and no further treatment was necessary.

In four patients shunt flow was reduced by hyperplastic intimal growth resulting in restenosis inside the vascular implant within three to six months after implantation. In all patients percutaneous removal of the hyperplastic intima was achieved. In eight of nine cases shunts are still open and used for hemodialysis.

Discussion

Percutaneous treatment of stenoses in hemodialysis fistulae has shown equal or even better results when compared to operative revision. But venous outflow stenoses in hemodialysis shunts are often very tight and may require high pressures during angioplasty. A considerable number of lesions do not respond well to simple balloon dilatation. There are other venous lesions which may be dilated easily but collapses immediately after dilatation. Both types of lesions will benefit by stent implantation, since the implant stabilizes the vascular wall and the continuous pressure of the self-expanding device maintains a dilating effect on the stenotic area [1-3].

In the early course a thrombogenic effect of the foreign body material has to be considered; later on the stent will be covered by neointima [1]. Intimal hyperplasia in the draining vein is a common problem in hemodialysis fistulae, which has been also found with venous stents. Due to hyperplastic intimal growth restenosis of the stent is a frequent sequelae especially in hemodialysis fistulae [2, 4], which may be treated percutaneously. Thus, careful follow-up is advisable in order to plan revision in time. Due to those restenoses, long-term results may appear less favorable [4]. But considering the fact that all procedures were performed in highly complicated cases, shunt function could be maintained in all patients and percutaneous revision was easy to perform. Thus, we think that stent implacement is indicated as an adjunct to balloon dilatation in cases of shunt stenoses or occlusions that do not respond well to balloon angioplasty alone, before operative revision is performed or new shunts are created.

References

[1] ROUSSEAU, H., J. PUEL, F. JOFFRE, et al.: Self-expanding endovascular prosthesis: an experimental study. *Radiology* 164: 709 (1987).

[2] GÜNTHER, R. W., D. VORWERK, K. BOHNDORF, et al.: Self-expanding metallic stent for the treatment of dialysis shunt stenoses. *Radiology* 170: 401 (1989).

[3] ZOLLIKOFER, C. L., I. LARGIADER, W. F. BRUHLMANN, et al.: Endovascular stenting of veins and grafts: preliminary clinical experience. *Radiology* 167: 707 (1988).

[4] JOFFRE, F., H. ROUSSEAU, J. PUECH, et al.: Treatment of hemodialysis arteriovenous fistula stenosis by percutaneous implantation of a new intravascular stent. VI. European Congress of Radiology 1987, 31.5.-6.6., Lisbon, Paper 0377.

Hemodialysis Catheters: Early Complications Related to Insertion Technique

R. PONIKVAR, A. KANDUS, J. DRINOVEC, M. MALOVRH, R. KVEDER, M. KAJTNA-KOSELJ, J. VARL, A. GUČEK, M. BENEDIK, A. BREN, A. SUHADOLNIK-LIČINA S. KAPLAN-PAVLOVČIČ, B. ČIŽMAN

Abstract

Twelve years experience with acute complications after insertion of 3240 femoral and 580 subclavian, a total of 3820 hemodialysis catheters is reviewed. The main complications were large hematomas after femoral catheters placement (1.5/1000) and pneumothorax, hematopneumothorax and mediastinal hematoma after subclavian vein cannulation (8.6/1000). All patients with acute complications survived.

Introduction

Large vein hemodialysis catheters have become the most popular acute vascular access in recent years [1]. They have been used for acute hemodialysis in patients with acute renal failure or acute poisoning, in patients who needed plasma exchange having had exhausted peripheral veins and in chronic hemodialysis patients who had been waiting for arterio-venous (A-V) fistula. A great advantage of hemodialysis catheters over A-V shunts and A-V fistulas is their rapid insertion and instantaneous possibility of applications. Insertion is quick, easy and safe when performed by experienced physicians but one must be aware of risks and even fatal complications [1-4].

The purpose of this paper is to report on acute serious complications related to insertion of femoral and subclavian hemodialysis catheters.

Material and Methods

Between April 1976 and June 1988 a total of 3820 hemodialysis (HD) catheters were placed either into femoral or subclavian vein. Catheters were used as a temporary vascular access for acute HD (patients with acute renal failure or acute intoxication), for plasma exchange and for chronic HD in patients without A-V fistula.

We used single lumen catheters, made of polyurethane or Teflon, lengths 12.5-25 cm, with internal diameter less than 2 mm. For subclavian vein cannulation catheters of 15 and 20 cm of length were used. The infraclavicular approach was used and the Seldinger insertion technique was applied.

Results

In the last 12 years a total of 3820 large vein HD catheters were placed, 3240 into femoral (84.82 %) and 580 into subclavian vein (15.18 %). Ten immediate serious complications were observed (2.6 per 1000 insertions), five after femoral (1.5 per 1000 insertions) and five after subclavian vein cannulation (8.6 per 1000 insertions).

Large subcutaneous, subfascial or retroperitoneal hematomas were leading complications after femoral catheters insertion. Local pain or abdominal discomfort, hypotension during HD and profound fall of hemoglobin concentration were the main clinical signs. In two patients of five the diagnosis of bleeding was confirmed by visible hematomas at puncture site having been spread subcutaneously towards the leg and thorax, in two ultrasound examination detected large retroperitoneal hematomas and in one a retroperitoneal hematoma was diagnosed some months later by autopsy. The site of bleeding was not detected by x-ray flebography (two patients), by arteriography (one patient) or by surgical exploration (one patient). In all patients catheters were removed at the beginning or during hemodialysis, compression of puncture site was performed and blood transfusion was given. No further complications were observed thereafter. Results are presented in Table 1.

Table 1. Immediate serious complications related to insertion of femoral HD catheters*.

No	Patient	Sex	Age	Underlying disease	Complication	Diagnostic procedure
1	E. H.	male	45	ESRD	retroperitoneal hematoma	x-ray flebography
2	M. J.	female	47	ESRD	subcutaneous, subfascial hematoma (leg, thorax)	clinical examination
3	J. B.	female	40	ESRD	subcutaneous hematoma (leg)	clinical examination
4	M. A.	female	60	ESRD	retroperitoneal hematoma	ultrasound, arteriography, surgical exploration
5	S. M.	female	10	ARF	retroperitoneal hematoma	flebography, ultrasound

* Outcome: All patients survived.

Pneumothorax or hematopneumothorax were the most common complications after subclavian vein cannulation. Out of five complicated catheter insertions we observed hematopneumothorax in two cases, pneumothorax in one, mediastinal hematoma in one and puncture of the trachea with dramatic but short lasting hemoptysis in one case. Diagnosis was established by clinical signs (chest pain, dyspnea) and chest x-ray examination. In all patients the catheter was immediately removed and compression of the puncture site was performed. Two patients were given blood transfusions and in one patient thoractic drainage was necessary. There were no further complications. Complications after subclavian catheters insertion are presented in Table 2.

Table 2. Immediate serious complications related to insertion of subclavian HD catheters.*

No	Patient	Sex	Age	Underlying disease	Complication	Therapeutic approach
1	S. K.	female	18	acute poisoning	hematopneumothorax	removal of the catheter
2	A. D.	female	72	ESRD	hematopneumothorax	removal of the catheter, thoracic drainage, blood transfusion
3	S. F.	female	24	ESRD	pneumothorax	removal of the catheter
4	K. B.	female	59	ESRD	mediastinal hematoma	removal of the catheter, blood transfusion
5	J. L.	female	50	ESRD	puncture of trachea	not necessary

* Outcome: All patients survived.

Discussion

Popularity of large vein catheters for HD is based on advantages such as easy placement and removal, reliability, relatively simple care and sparing of peripheral veins. On the other side there is a threat of complications which may be even fatal. Many of complications are related to the technique of insertion [5].

Major complication after insertion of 3240 HD femoral catheters was large hematoma, either subfascial and subcutaneous or retroperitoneal. Rate of complications was low (1.5/1000 insertions). In all cases puncture of the femoral artery or repeated puncture of the femoral veins with the insertion needle resulted in prolonged bleeding because of preexistent hemostatic disorders. Firm compression of the puncture site is of great value. Surgical intervention is rarely necessary while symptomatic therapy and medical survey should be carried out with great care.

Rate of complications after insertion of 580 subclavian HD catheters is higher than for femoral ones but relatively low (8.6/1000 insertions) compared to the literature [2-4, 6, 7]. The main cause of our complications reviewed was mechanical trauma of pleura or/and subclavian artery. Both were probably due to the relative lack of skill and experience of insertion technique. Careful symptomatic treatment was carried out in all patients and in only one thoracic drainage was necessary.

Conclusions

Our 12 years experience with 3820 femoral and subclavian hemodialysis catheters confirmed popularity of this type of acute vascular access.

The rate of acute serious complications after insertion was only 2.6/1000 insertions related to 3820 cannulations of femoral and subclavian veins. We had no fatal complications.

References

[1] LAL, S. M., D. FOWLER, D. PHILLIPS, T. LILLICK, G. G. BERG, R. KHANNA: Internal jugular vein thrombosis after subclavian vein cannulation: detection by computed tomography. *Int. J. Artif. Organs* 9: 251-252 (1986).

[2] FINE, A., D. CHURCHILL, H. GAULT, G. MATHIESON: Fatality due to subclavian dialysis catheter. *Nephron* 29: 99-100 (1981).

[3] ERBEN, J., J. KVASNICKA, J. BASTECKY, J. GROH, J. ZAHRADNIK, V. ROZSIVAL, D. BASTEEKA, P. FIXA, J. KOZAK, V. HEROUT: Long-term experience with the technique of subclavian and femoral vein cannulation in hemodialysis. *Art. Organs* 3: 241-244 (1979).

[4] WALDMAN, R. P., M. DONNER, A. C. BILSKY, M. C. STOM, R. G. NARINS: Delayed onset of hemothorax: an unusual complication of subclavian access for hemodialysis. *Nephron* 37: 270-272 (1984).

[5] HICKMANN, R. O., S. WATKINS: A review of hemodialysis catheters and access devices. *Dialysis and Transplantation* 16: 481-486 (1987).

[6] VAZIRI, N. D., M. MAKSY, M. LEWIS, D. MARTIN, K. EDWARDS: Massive mediastinal hematoma caused by a double lumen subclavian catheter. *Art. Organs* 8: 223-226 (1984).

[7] HANSBROUGH, J. F., J. A. NARROD, G. V. STIEGMAN: Cardiac perforation and tamponade from malpositioned subclavian dialysis catheter. *Nephron* 32: 363-364 (1982).

Percutaneous Transluminal Angioplasty in the Treatment of Renal Transplant Artery Stenosis

J.-D. Lian, C.-H. Cheng

Abstract

Renal transplant artery stenosis occurred in seven patients of 73 cadaver renal transplants during a five-year period at Taichung Veterans General Hospital.

Post-transplant hypertension with or without deterioration of renal function were noted clinically. Percutaneous transluminal angioplasty was performed in five patients. Four of them had dramatic clinical improvement, only one failed due to arterial spasm during percutaneous transluminal angioplasty.

We conclude that acute rejection may resemble renal artery stenosis in patients presented mainly with declining renal function. In such patients early diagnosis and treatment of renal transplant artery stenosis with percutaneous transluminal angioplasty can reserve normal renal graft function.

Introduction

Renal transplant artery stenosis (RTAS) is one of the major causes of post-transplantation hypertension. Before percutaneous transluminal angioplasty (PTA) was introduced [1], surgical repairment is the major procedure of management. However surgical treatment has a significant risk of mortality and morbidity. Percutaneous transluminal angioplasty is an alternative and probably a safer treatment modality in RTAS [2-6].

Because of limited cases published, we add our experiences of PTA in six patients with renal transplant artery stenosis.

Material and Methods

From 1982 to 1988, 73 cases of cadaveric renal transplants were performed in our hospital. Transplant renal artery stenosis was diagnosised in seven patients by angiography. They all underwent end-to-end anastomosis with donor renal artery to internal iliac artery of the recipient. All seven patients received prednisolone and cyclosporin for immunosuppression. The cyclosporin dosage was adjusted to keep a plasma level between 50 to 150 ng/ml. After RTAS was confirmed, six of the seven patients underwent percutaneous transluminal angioplasty. The seventh patient refused the procedure. PTA was performed using a balloon and a dilutation catheter (Cook Inc., Bloomington, Indiana, USA). The size of the catheter and the lengths of balloon was selected appropriate for the patients with different lengths and sizes of stenosis. The catheter was inserted percutaneously into the femoral artery by the Seldinger technique and forwarded to the site of the stenosis. The balloon was kept distended for 15 seconds at the recommended pressure. After successful angioplasty low dosage of heparin (2000-5000 U) was given intravenously with antiplatelet agents.

Results

Seven patients out of 73 patients developed RTAS. The incidence was 9.6 %. Six patients received percutaneous transluminal angioplasty. PTA was successful in five patients, with only one failure (case 2) due to arterial spasm. The arterial spasm was irreversible, in spite of intensive therapy with intravenous nitroglycerin and streptokinase infusion.

Blood pressure, creatinine and site of stenosis are shown in Table 1. Three patients had stenosis at the anastomosis site and the other four patients had stenosis distal to the anastomosis. The interval between transplantation and the diagnosis of RTAS ranged from four to six months.

Four of the six cases improved their graft function after PTA, the serum creatinine dropped dramatically after the procedure. Although the difference was not statistically significant, these four patients were able to keep a stable renal function for a follow up duration from 10 to 34 months. Hypertension was dramatically improved in case 5 after successful angioplasty and was stable for a follow up of one year.

Discussion

Percutaneous transluminal angioplasty was first introduced for treatment of coronary artery disease. The pathology of coronary artery disease was mainly due to atherosclerotic plaque. The mechanisms of PTA in atherosclerotic disease had been studied thoroughly. It was believed that PTA causes disruption and splitting of the atherosclerotic plaque and stretching of the outer elastic media and adventitia, which in turn resulted in enlargement of the lumen. Percutaneous transluminal angioplasty (PTA) was introduced for treating RTAS since 1979 [3]. The pathology of this non-atherosclerosis stenosis was variable from fibrous endarteritis to intimal thickening. The mechanism of PTA in treatment of renal transplant artery stenosis is poorly understood. Chandrasoma [4] reported a high failure rate of PTA in treatment of RTAS located at the anastomotic site. Pathological finding of stenosis

Table 1. Clinical Data and Results of Percutaneous Transluminal Angioplasty in Renal Transplant Artery Stenosis.

Case	Age/Sex	Original Disease	Sites of Stenosis	Before PTA Cr (mg%)	BP (mmHg)	After PTA Cr (mg%)	BP (mmHg)	Comment
1.	44/M	Chronic nephritis	75 % Anastomosis	6.5	157/95	1.9	150/90	Successful PTA Follow up 16 months
2.	40/M	Glomerulonephritis	75 % Distal to anastomosis	8.6	138/84	–	–	Renal artery spasm results in graft lost
3.	25/M	Glomerulonephritis	75 % Anastomosis	4.2	154/90	3.4	132/79	Successful PTA Graft lost due to chronic rejection and UT1 2 years later
4.	25/F	IgA nephropathy	75 % Anastomosis	6.4	139/88	3.7	149/96	Successful PTA Follow up 10 months
5.	25/F	Glomerulonephritis	75 % Distal to anastomosis	3.14	155/90	2.8	130/78	Successful PTA Follow up 34 months
6.	34/M	Glomerulonephritis	80 % Distal to anastomosis	3.8	166/104	3.4	124/83	Successful PTA follow up 28 months
7.	49/M	Chronic nephritis	50 % Distal to anastomosis	2.6	172/128	–	–	Patient refused angioplasty and expired 3 months later

at the anastomotic site showed nodular fibrotic lesion with calcification. He believed that surgical repair is the treatment of choice in these patients. Recurrent stenosis is a problem of angioplasty. Although the successful rate of PTA treatment in RTAS is high, the incidence of restenosis is still unknown. The five patients who successfully relieved their stenosis remained patent for 10 to 34 months during follow-up. Although no restenosis was observed, it is still too early, to make any conclusion and long term followed up is needed.

Recently repeated PTA in treatment of coronary heart disease had a high success rate in Cleveland Clinic. Third PTA has also been introduced. It would be expected that the same result can be seen in the treatment of restenosis in RTAS.

Complications of percutaneous transluminal angioplasty is not uncommon. There had been reports of perforation of renal artery at anastomosis, renal artery spasm and renal artery thrombosis [3, 6-8]. In our patient 2, irreversible renal artery spasm resulted in renal graft loss. We suggest good preparation and skillful management of the procedure be carried out to reduce the incidence of complication.

In a literature review from Lohr [9], PTA had a lower mortality rate and safer method than surgical treatment. We agree that PTA should be the first choice of management in patients with RTAS.

References

[1] Diamond, N. G., W. J. Casarella, M. A. Hardy, G. B. Appel: Dilatation of critical transplant renal artery stenosis by percutaneous transluminal angioplasty. *AJR* 133: 1167-1169 (1979).

[2] Carr, D., R. O. Quin, D. H. N. Hamilton, J. D. Briggs, B. J. R. Junor, P. F. Semple: Transluminal dilatation of transplant renal artery stenosis. *BMJ* 1: 196-197 (1980).

[3] Sindermann, K. W., S. Sprayregen, T. A. Sos, et al.: Percutaneous transluminal dilatation in renal transplant arterial stenosis. *Transplantation* 30: 400-444 (1980).

[4] Chandrasoma, A. M. Aberle: Anastomotic line renal artery stenosis after transplantation. *J. Urology* 135: 1159-1162 (1986).

[5] Grossmann, R. A., D. C. Dafoe, R. B. Shoenfield, et al.: Percutaneous transluminal angioplasty treatment of renal artery stenosis. *Transplantation* 34: 339-343 (1982).

[6] Greenstein, S. M., A. Verstandig, G. K. Molean, et al.: Percutaneous transluminal angioplasty. *Transplantation* 43: 29-31 (1987).

[7] Lohr, J. W., M. L. Macdougall, A. M. Chonko, et al.: Percutaneous transluminal angioplasty in transplant renal artery stenosis: experience and review of literature. *Am. J. Kidney Dis.* 7: 363-367 (1986).

[8] Mahler, F., J. Triller, P. Weidmann, B. Nachbur: Complication in percutaneous transluminal dilatation of renal arteries. *Nephron* 44: Suppl. 1: 63-66 (1986).

[9] Lohr, J. W., M. L. Macdougall, A. M. Chonko, D. A. Diederich, et al.: Percutaneous transluminal angioplasty in transplant artery experience and review of the literature. *Am. J. Kidney Dis.* 7: 363-367 (1986).

Doppler Velocity Measurements: Adequate Noninvasive Test Assessing the Capacity of Arteriovenous Fistulas for Chronic Hemodialysis?

M. MALOVRH, A. GUČEK, B. ČIŽMAN, J. DRINOVEC

Abstract

Doppler velocity measurements as a noninvasive test for assessing the capacity of an arteriovenous fistula (AVF) for chronic hemodialysis has been developed. The test is based on transcutaneous Doppler measurements of the brachial artery before and after compression of the venous part of the AVF. The velocity index is calculated. The velocity index of three or more is always associated with sufficient AVF capacity. This test is also useful for control AVF postoperatively and to assess fistula maturation.

Introduction

Angioaccess is the most important determinant for the continuous well-being of patients with end stage renal disease who are supported on hemodialysis [1, 2]. A direct internal arteriovenous fistula (AVF) is the procedure of choice and provides the best possible blood access. The total fistula flow must be at least 300 ml/min, preferably between 400 and 800 ml/min [1, 2]. Assessment of the AVF capacity can be done by different methods. Doppler velocity measurements (DV) as noninvasive test to assess fistula capacity is reported [3].

Patients and Methods

We examined 27 patients with surgically constructed AVF in the arm with an anastomosis between the end of the cephalic vein and the side of the radial artery. 27 patients, age between 23 and 74 years, with an average age (± SD) of 50.8 (±12.6) years had been treated with chronic hemodialysis (HD) from 0.5 to 75 months, mean 24.9 months. DV were performed on the brachial artery of the fistula side before and after compression at the venous part of the AVF. The velocity before compression (Vo) divided by the velocity after compression (Vc) is the velocity index (Vi).

For DV the bidirectional Doppler apparatus with transducer at 8 MHz (Vasoflo 2 Sonicaid, Chicester, England) was used. The angle between the Doppler transducer and the brachial artery was fixed at 45° with a plastic holder for the transducer. In order to establish the value of DV the maximal useful fistula flow (MUFF) was measured during HD with the Fistula Assessment Monitor Gambro FAM 10-1 (Gambro, Sweden). Maximal blood flow that could be measured was limited to 500 ml/min.

A second group of nine patients, aged 24 to 74 years (mean age 51.9 years) was followed before and after construction of the AVF. These patients were not on chronic HD yet. The first DV were done before, and then on the 7th and 14th day after construction, four weeks, and three months later.

The Student t-test for paired data was used for the comparison of pre- and postoperative values of Vi. The correlation coefficient by Pearson was calculated to establish the relationship between the Vi and the MUFF.

Results

Velocity index (mean ± SD) in 27 patients was 6.7 ± 4.1, ranging from 1.6 to 14.5. 21 AVFs had an index of 3 or more, four AVFs had an index between 2.1 and 2.8, and two AVFs less than two. MUFF in twenty-two AVFs was between 400 and 500 ml/min, in three cases between 300 and 400 ml/min, and two AVFs had MUFF less than 200 ml/min. There was only one false negative result, when Vi of less than three was calculated and MUFF 450 ml/min was measured. The relationship between Vi and MUFF is shown in Figure 1. Correlation coefficient is 0.45 ($p < 0.05$). The sensitivity of this test is 95.5 %, and specificity 100 %.

In the second group of patients, Vi was higher than the initial immediately after construction of the AVF ($p < 0.01$). The final and stable fistula capacity was found between two and four weeks after construction (Table 1).

Table 1. Velocity index before and after construction of the arteriovenous fistula (n = 9).

Number of patient	Before Operation	7th day	14th day	4 weeks	3 months
1	1.3	2.1^+	3.2	4.9	10.2
2*	1.2	1.7^+	2.4	2.1	2.3
3	1.8	2.2^+	4.8	7.2	8.3
4	2.0	2.3^+	3.5	4.3	11.0
5	1.7	2.0^+	3.8	7.2	–
6	1.9	2.5^+	3.1	8.9	–
7	1.4	1.9^+	2.8	3.5	–
8	1.2	1.8^+	2.2	–	–
9	1.1	2.0^+	2.5	5.4	–

* maximal useful fistula flow during hemodialysis 450 ml/min.
$^+$ $p < 0.01$.

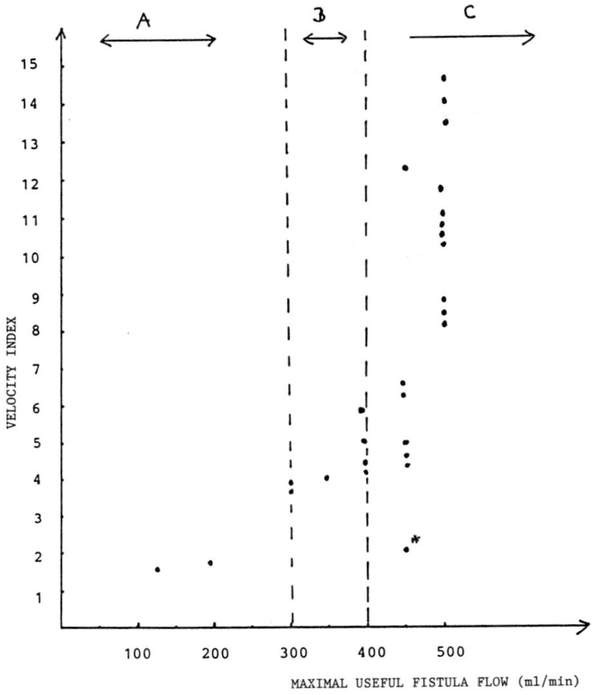

Fig. 1. The relationship between the velocity index and maximal useful fistula flow (A: poorly functioning fistula, B: moderately functioning fistula, C: well functioning fistula).

Discussion

Blood velocity at any given instant is determined by the ratio of blood pressure over peripheral resistance [4, 5]. Peripheral resistance is determined by the presence or absence of obstruction in the pathway. Vasoconstriction can mimic the effect of distal peripheral obstruction. In the case of AVF, compression of the venous part of AVF can mimic vasoconstriction, and the velocity over the brachial artery is diminished. The velocity obtained during undisturbed flow (Vo) divided by that obtained during compression of the efferent part of the AVF (Vc) is the velocity index (Vo/Vc). The greater is AVF capacity the greater is Vi [4]. In our study, velocity index of three or more was always associated with adequate extracorporeal dialysis blood flow.

In conclusions, DV as a noninvasive test to assess fistula capacity is very useful. This method can immediately clarify whether the cause of poor extracorporeal blood flow is poor AVF capacity or an inadequate needle placement, and so this test may also result in better directed operations. The frequency of fistula angiography can be reduced. This noninvasive test is also very useful to control AVF postoperatively and to assess fistula maturation.

References

[1] DRINOVEC, J., N. VODOPIJA, T. DARIJAN, S. LUZAR, J. SIMONITI: Pristup krvnim sudovima za hemodializu, pp. 124-135. In: JOVANOVIC, V. (ed.): Uremija. Medicinska knjiga: Zagreb 1976.

[2] BUTT, K. M. H.: Angioaccess. In: DRUKKER, W., F. M. PARSON, J. F. MAHER (eds.): Replacement of renal function by dialysis. Boston, Martinus Nijhoff Publishers, 171-185 (1983).

[3] RUTHERFORD, R. B.: Noninvasive testing in the diagnosis and assessment of arteriovenous fistula, pp. 430-442. In: BERNSTEIN, E. F. (ed.): Noninvasive diagnostic techniques in vascular disease. The C. V. Mosby Company: St. Louis 1982.

[4] SHOOR, P. M., A. FRONEK, E. F. BERNSTEIN: Current instrumentation for Doppler velocity studies, pp. 22-26. In: BERNSTEIN, E. F. (ed.): Noninvasive diagnostic techniques in vascular disease. The C. V. Mosby Company: St. Louis 1982.

[5] STRADNESS, D. E.: Doppler ultrasonic techniques in vascular disease, pp. 13-21. In: BERNSTEIN, E. F. (ed.): Noninvasive diagnostic techniques in vascular disease. The C. V. Mosby Company: St. Louis 1982.

Percutaneous Transluminal Angioplasty Versus Surgery

B. Kramann, K. Scherer

Abstract

From January 1984 to August 1988 we performed 162 percutaneous transluminal angioplasties (PTA) in 147 patients. The lesions were localized as shown in Table 1.

Table 1. Localization of lesions.

Iliacal stenoses	n = 94	(58.0%)
Femoral stenoses	n = 25	(15.5%)
Femoral occlusions	n = 24	(14.8%)
Popliteal stenoses	n = 9	(5.6%)
Popliteal occlusions	n = 7	(4.3%)
Occlusions of distal arteries	n = 3	(1.8%)

43.9 % of the cases presented iliac stenoses alone, in 31.8 % there were only stenoses and/or occlusions in the femoropopliteal region. In 22.5 % the patients suffered from multiple lesions in more than one region. The patient's mean age was 59.8 ± 9.3 years, 85.7 % were male, 14.3 % were female.

Before intervention 16.7 % of the patients presented clinical stage IIa, 63.5 % stage IIb, 8.3 % stage III and 11.5 % stage IV.

Table 2. Risk factors.

Smoking	(56.4%)
Hypertonus	(17.2%)
Hyperlipidemia	(16.4%)
Diabetes	(10.0%)

The risk factors are listed in Table 2. In 70 % there was only one risk factor, in 14.3 % of the patients presented two and in 3.5 % three risk factors. In three patients the transaxillary approach was necessary. In 21 patients the PTA was combined with local infusion of 100,000 U of urokinase. The criteria for the assessment of the postinterventional results were as follows:

- Treated segment patent or residual stenosis < 50 %.
- Improvement of clinical stage for at least one stage.
- Raise of doppler ratio by at least 0.2.

The overall primary success rate was 93.0 %. In the iliac lesions it was 95.5 %, the success rate of femoropopliteal lesions was 84.6 %. The long term results are shown in Table 3:

Table 3. Cumulative patency rate, life table method.

	n	6 mths	12 mths	24 mths	36 mths	48 mths
Iliac stenoses alone	69	98.4	95.5	90.7	84.1	84.1
Stenoses and occlusions femoropopliteal	48	89.7	81.9	81.9	81.9	81.9
Lesions in more than one region	34	87.3	80.2	75.4	67.1	53.7

The rate of complications which required surgery was 2.5 %.

The results of our interventions are consistent with those reported in the literature. The primary success rate in the iliac segment is > 90 %, the success rate of the femoropopliteal segment is reported to range between 50 to 90 %.

The long term results in the mostly inhomogenous patient groups are in a large scattering range depending on age, clinical stage, localization and length of the lesion. In the isolated iliac, stenosis patency rates of 80 % after five years are common. In the femoropopliteal segment the five years patency rate varies between 20 and 85 %.

Up to now there is no prospective randomized study on PTA versus surgery. A comparison between the reported results of surgery and of PTA is difficult because of the existence of numerous variables and their lack of standardization. However, it appears that the long term patency of saphenous grafts is slightly superior to the results after angioplasty while PTA is superior to bypass grafts performed with any other material.

Furthermore, repeated PTA is easier to perform than surgical repair of grafts. Additionally PTA allows us to preserve saphenous veins for coronary or carotid surgery if necessary.

Peritoneal Access: Overview

Methods and Technology in Peritoneal Dialysis

P. R. VERREET

Abstract

The different materials used for catheters in peritoneal dialysis are briefly discussed and the implantation techniques are outlined. The total number of 122 primary implantations between 1979 and 1989 at the University of Düsseldorf are separated into different time periods and it is shown the decrease of nonmetabolic complications after introducing a standardized implantation technique. In the discussion is pointed out that the continuous ambulatory peritoneal dialysis may be improved by modifications of the existing implants and by further standardization of the implantation technique – a task for technology and surgery.

Introduction

A low risk access to the abdominal cavity via an implanted catheter is the key to successful peritoneal dialysis. The introduction and spread of continuous ambulatory peritoneal dialysis (CAPD) on an outpatient basis was followed by an increased demand for better catheter equipment.

Since Palmer and his coworkers designed the first silicone catheter for the purpose of peritoneal dialysis, a lot of different catheter models were produced, which shows that the procedure has not been optimized so far.

Up to date there is still a high rate of non metabolic catheter dependent complications. This has brought us to reevaluate the whole concept of catheter design.

Catheters and Methods

We believe that one of the main shortcomings in traditional catheter constructions lies in the choice of materials used (Table 1). The lack of elasticity excluded polyethylene for continuous use in peritoneal dialysis although it had been used in peritoneal lavage catheters. The same applies for PVC which proved to be too hard a substance to be permanently implanted in the abdominal wall.

Silicone has found widespread acceptance and has been used as the basic substance for all varieties of catheters. It is characterized by an acceptable degree of

Table 1. Characterization of Polymers for Medical Use (e.g. CAPD-Catheter).

Polyethylene (PE)	Molecular weight up to 10^6, soft elastic polymers, inert, smooth surface, thermoplastic, no rubber elasticity, processing without additives.
Polyvinylchloride (PVC)	Hard, thermoplastic material, softeners (40 %) and stabilisators (UV, radical-protective substances) improve the workability, elastic, adhesive.
Silicone (Sil)	"cold polymerization" in polysiloxane with tetrabutyltitanate (silanol ends); "hot polymerization" in polysiloxanes with peroxydes, (integrated vinyl groups); siliciumoxyd as filling material, removal of additional substances by elution with water and consecutive boiling.
Polyurethane (PUR)	Soft to rigid polymere (variation of Diisocynate + Diol) soluble, thermoplastic, no additives, no stabilizers, purity by dissolution, precipitation.

elasticity and has proved to be almost biologically inert. However the workability of silicone is not yet optimized as is seen in the roughness of this catheter's perforation.

Since the development of laminated polyurethane the elasticity can be varied to high degree by adding soft or hard segment substrates at variable proportions. Moreover when medically used it has proven to be absolutely inert. Another advantage besides the variability of elasticity is the fact that for example catheter perforation can be added as smooth as the rest of the catheter surface.

If one considers the elastic features of the previously mentioned materials, one realizes that polyethylene and PVC are too rigid to be used as permanent catheter implants. In the stress strain behavior (Fig. 1) silicone and polyurethane seem to be of equal elasticity, but as already mentioned the elasticity of polyurethane is variable and can be adjusted accordingly.

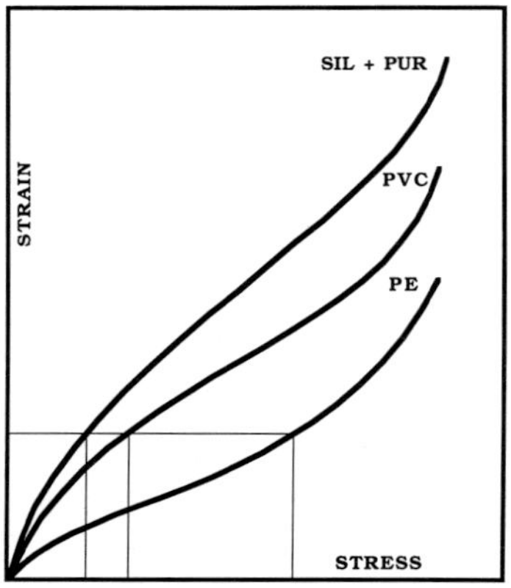

Fig. 1. Stress-strain behavior of common catheter materials.

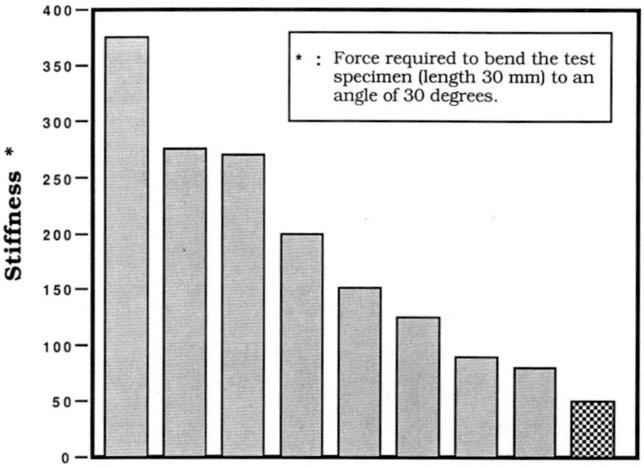

Fig. 2. Stiffness of different catheters.

A list of the tested stiffness of all CAPD catheter models produced is presented in Figure 2. The first three catheters are made of polyethylene and PVC. The rest are silicone catheters and the last model has gone into production recently to be available at the end of this year. Its basic matrix is polyurethane which has been modified according to detailed conceptions with regard to the production of a permanent peritoneal catheter.

Regarding the biocompatibility of materials for medical use we briefly present a test according to Lowrey, which is commonly used to examine biocompatibility. It is based on the quantification of growth inhibition of fibroplasts by estimating the protein-contents of the environment after the exposure to different testing materials. As Table 2 shows the first two substances cause a total growth inhibition whereas silicone and polyurethane provoke a minimal reduction in fibroplast activity only.

Table 2. Biocompatibility Test.

Test material	Growth inhibition (in %)*
Bard Biocath	100
Silkolatex R.-G.	100
Argyle Silicone	3
PUR-Tube	3

*Growth inhibition test with L-929 fibroblasts and measurement of protein content according to Lowrey (2 cm^2/ml).

Table 3. Comparison of Catheter Materials.

	Elasticity	Workability	Biocompatibility	Price
PE	–	○–	○	+
PVC	○–	+	– –	+
SIL	+	–	+	–
PUR	+	+	+	○

The final evaluation of all substances with regard to elasticity, workability, biocompatibility and last but not least costs (Table 3) shows polyurethane as the material with most technical advantages with the exception of the higher price. The main disadvantage of silicone remains that the workability of this material is limited as we discussed earlier.

We will refrain from criticizing all different varieties of catheters by pointing out the chemical and physical features of the materials used. We would just like to point out that advantageous material properties of commonly used implants are not yet sufficiently utilized. This applies to surface properties, elastic behavior, biostability and biocompatibility.

But finally let us discuss about the actual implants for medical use. Some centers still use trocar implantation even for continuous peritoneal dialysis. Little is being published but studies from Canada and Italy show a considerably higher complication rate as would be expected with surgical implantation.

In use are double cuff and single cuff catheters in the original form, the common Tenckhoff-catheters, and a modification with a pigtail which again is available with one or two cuffs. Silicone catheters are supplied with a Dacron felt cuff which is brought into position into the abdominal wall. Dacron felt cuffs are supposed to provoke a foreign body reaction which again causes granulomatous reactions in the surrounding tissues and thus are supposed to protect the catheter tunnel. Dacron felt is a suitable material because it has an increased exposed surface due to the foaming of the material during the manufacture. Furthermore it is a material of low biological inerture which induces an extensive foreign body reaction once it is implanted. The pigtail prevents any obstruction of influx and efflux of dialysate by approximated coils of gut. It also supplies the catheter with certain positional stability with the abdominal cavity.

In the transrectal implantation the catheter goes through the abdominal wall. The innermost Dacron felt cuff comes to lie epiperitoneal whereas the outer cuff lies in the subcutaneous layer. The course of the catheter is relatively straight and stretched. One can imagine how a reduction of the abdominal wall for instance by weight loss may provoke a protrusion of the outer cuff.

Another model of a silicone catheter is supplied with an umbrella of Goretex. The Goretex umbrella comes to lie within the abdominal wall that the collar comes into position immediately subcutaneously and the covering runs through the whole length of the abdominal wall, for example in a transrectal implantation.

The catheter model most commonly used is probably the Toronto Western Hospital catheter according to Oreopulos-Zellermann. It is also made of silicone, but has certain advantages compared to the other models (Table 4). The course through the abdominal wall is again secured by two Dacron felt cuffs, but the pass point through the peritoneum is supplied with a silicone ball which is faced to a Dacron felt plate to prevent leakage. Two silicone plates attached to the intraabdominal part of the catheter will prevent dislocation quite sufficiently. The catheter shows perforations over almost the whole intraabdominal segment. The plates that protect the transrectal implanted catheter against dislocation come to lie approximately to the Douglas pouch. The point of passing through the peritoneal layer is sealed with a Dacron-disc faced to the silicone ball and the catheter itself describes a soft curved way through the muscle and the subcutaneous layer.

This kind of implantation technique which we have practiced since 1983 is demonstrated. The procedure is carried out in general anesthesia. The main advantage is the relaxation of the abdominal wall which makes a primary water

Table 4. Technical Evaluation of CAPD Catheters.

	Oreopoulus Zellermann	Gore	Swan-Neck
Material	Silicone Elastomer	Silicone Elastomer	Silicone Elastomer
Internal Diameter	2.8 mm	2.7 mm	2.9 mm
Outer Diameter	5.1 mm	4.9 mm	4.9 mm
Wall Thickness	1.15 mm	1.1 mm	1.0 mm
Tensile Test Standard Deviation	10.1 N 0.3 N	9.9 N 0.3 N	8.2 N 0.2 N
Bending Test Standard Deviation	0.83 N 0.02 N	0.54 N 0.02 N	0.46 N 0.03 N
The tests have been carried out on a 50 N "Zwick" universal tester. Test length: 50 mm; Elongation: 100 %; Speed of elongation: 100 mm/min.			
The bending tests have been carried out on a Frank rigidity tester. Test length: 10 mm; Angle of deflection: 30°.			

tight closure of the abdomen possible. We choose the left lower abdomen as side of implantation to be able to place the intraabdominal course of the catheter at the left side of the mesenterial axis up to the Douglas pouch so that any dislocation at the implants end out of the Douglas pouch by movements of the intestine is prevented. We choose the transrectal approach. This way we can use the rectus abdomenis muscle as well vascularized covering of the catheter course. The cranio-caudal-incision is approximately 6 cm long.

After opening and inspection of the abdominal cavity the tip of the catheter is ventrally of the promontory advanced to the Douglas pouch under visual control. Again adequate exposure is only possible on the conditions of relaxation in general anesthesia.

The closure of the abdomen starts with a continuous water tight peritoneal suture which includes the given catheter segment in the distal wound angle. The catheter itself has to be fastened tightly with a monophile resorbable suture. After a tight peritoneal closure the external end of the catheter is pulled through a separate stab incision far away from the implantation wound. Therefore the catheter is armed with a guide pin. The stab incision is carried out in such a way that the catheter comes to lie in a wide curve without acute angle. The catheter is furthermore placed to the rectus abdominis muscle as well vascularized and flexible covering. The incision size is to perform in that way that the skin encloses the implant firmly but without tension.

As soon as the catheter is brought into its final position the external opening is connected to the system and a first flow trial can be observed.

We apply 500 ml of dialyzing fluid into the abdominal cavity to test the water tightness of the peritoneal suture. After this we close the wound in layers. The peritoneal dialysis has thus already started with a reduced volume of 500 ml of dialyzing fluid. It is worth mentioning that the catheter is radiopaque to identify any misplacement radiologically.

Results

We used this technique in our center since 1983. Before the implantation technique has not been standardized. The number of primary implantations performed at the department of surgery at the University of Düsseldorf per month is shown in Table 5. The continuous increase of implantations might show that this procedure has gained a certain popularity in the Federal Republic of Germany.

Table 5. CAPD Catheter Implantations. Operation Statistics I/1979 – IV/1988, Surgical Department at University of Düsseldorf, FRG.

implantation period	I/79-VI/83		VII/83-XII/86		I/87-XII/87		I/88-IV/88		Total	
new implantations	52		38		19		13		122	
complications	N	%	N	%	N	%	N	%	N	%
catheter dislocation	8	15.4	1	2.6	–	0.0	–	0.0	9	7.4
leakage	7	13.5	1	2.6	–	0.0	–	0.0	8	6.6
tunnel infection	12	23.1	7	18.4	2	10.5	1	7.7	21	17.2
peritonitis	19	36.5	8	21.1	2	5.3	1	7.7	29	23.8

Yet so far only 4 % of all patients with terminal renal insufficiency are treated with CAPD, while in the USA, Canada, Italy and Spain the proportion of peritoneal dialysis is considerably higher.

While our patient collective initially was mainly made up of patients with severe vascular access problems, diabetis mellitus and hydrophic cardiac insuffiency, we are nowadays faced to an increased demand by the patients themselves who have chosen this form of dialysis. Without such a negative patient selection the list of nonmetabolic complications could decrease furthermore.

Table 5 shows the total number of 122 primary implantations between 1979 and 1988 separated into different periods. The first period till June 1983 covers the time where we implanted different catheter models with different techniques. As we have already mentioned we have standardized the technique with the introduction of the Oreopoulos-Zellermann-catheter in July 1983. The period is listed beginning January 1987 to 1988 separately from the rest to show the decrease of nonmetabolic methodological complications which are listed in Table 5 too. Catheter dislocation it's to say the intraabdominal malposition of the catheter has disappeared completely. We believe this is due to the antidislocation features of the Oreopoulos-Zellermann-catheter. We have furthermore not had any more cases of leakage with fistula formation at the side where the catheter passes through the peritoneum. This may be explained by a modified suture technique under general anesthesia with a relaxed abdominal wall.

The intraoperative test for water tightness seems to be also quite important to be able to place correcting sutures at leaking sides.

The main remaining complications are on the one hand the so called tunnel infection and on the other hand peritonitis as major complications of peritoneal dialysis.

Exit site infections certainly make possible tunnel infections through the subcutaneous tissue into the deeper wall layers. This way even generalized peritonitis may be introduced. The exit site infection can be caused by a cuff protrusion through inadequate positioning of the external Dacron felt cuff at the time of implantation. In rare cases cuff prolaps can be induced by weight reduction A persisting site infection is typically surrounded by hypertrophic granulation tissue. Again this system has not been implanted correctly. The exit site position was chosen too close to the abdominal access.

Discussion

Aim of implantation is to place the intraabdominal catheter tip exactly to the Douglas pouch to drain the dialysis fluid almost completely. The course of the catheter at the abdominal wall should be without any tension to the surrounding tissue to avoid any cellular reaction. The fact is that it can only be achieved when the stiffness of the catheter permits a sufficient curvation and flexibility without impairment of the lumen. This is only a question of the implants working up depending mainly on material features.

In actual use silicone catheters elasticity is not sufficiently given to prevent certain pressure areas in the tunnel. Even correct implantation may not prevent a so called tunnel-decubitus which will show up in the subcutaneous course at any pressurized side cellular demarcation. The histological finding causes us to call for new implants without any spring back force as in common silicone catheters.

Tunnel decubitus presents primarly aseptic inflamatory reaction of the surrounding tissue. Macroscopically a fine film of fluid is filling out the tunnel which again may possibly be colonized and eventually develop a full blown tunnel infection with associated tissue reaction. It is understandable that – once this area has been passed the subcutaneous tunnel region by an infection – it may spread along the tunnel into the abdomen and cause a generalized peritonitis.

We would like to briefly mention an observation which we had made immediately after implantation of CAPD-catheters. The CAPD-peritonitis certainly presents a special form of peritonitis. It is – so to say – a peritonitis which is already being treated since according to surgical management one would irrigate and drain the abdomen. It is therefore understandable that in patients with CAPD-peritonitis the typical symptoms and signs of peritonitis are usually quite extenuated. After implantation of the system there will nevertheless be a definite increase of white cell count in dialysate fluid within the first week. This presents a sterile peritonitis since even with extensive attempts at isolating a contamination no pathogenic organism can be discovered. It may represent a cellular reaction to the implantation trauma or to the implanted catheter or the first contact with introduced dialysing fluid.

On the contrary there are of course cases of septic peritonitis either caused by continuous spread via a tunnel infection yet more commonly a result of contamination during dialysate changement. A consequent treatment of any exit site infection is important to prevent tunnel infection and finally peritonitis. It is of course a pre-condition for peritoneal dialysis that patients are adequately trained to avoid any peritoneal contamination.

The following can develop out of a septic peritonitis. A thin film of proteins covers the intraabdominal part of the catheter, mainly fibronectins. After contamination there may be a bacterial microcolonisation which is able to spread all over the catheters surface. By production of an extracellular polysaccharide substance the Kokkal-colonies produce a glucoconjugate possibly influenced by the presence of high sugar levels in the dialysate fluid. This makes the microorganism less succeptable to opsonisation and phagocytosis as well as for antibiotic treatment.

Finally we would like to point out that abdominal surgery is also possible in CAPD-patients. Table 6 lists the operations performed. They range from hernial repairs up to operations including gastro-intestinal anastomoses. It is remarkable that in all patients discussed here the peritoneal dialysis could be continued immediately after operation although in individual cases it had to be modified.

Table 6. Surgery in CAPD-Patients.

Herniotomy	10
Renal Transplantation	9
Abscess incision	3
Explorative laparotomy	2
Colonic resection	1
Partial gastric resection	1

In conclusion we can say that in spite of our limited experience with the peritoneal dialysis in West Germany we may predict a future for this method which may be improved by modifications of the existing implants and by standardization of the implantation technique. This is a task for technology and surgery which will finally allows nephrologists to use CAPD without problems.

Closed CAPD: A New System to Reduce Peritonitis Risk in CAPD

A. Berke

Abstract

A newly developed sterile connecting device for CAPD is presented. This system allows for the first time in CAPD to perform the change of solution bags in a closed system. This principle avoids bacterial contamination and a break-through in the reduction of peritonitis risk is achieved. It can be speculated that this system will help CAPD to gain a bigger share in the treatment of dialysis patients.

Introduction

CAPD has proven to be effective in the treatment of patients with terminal kidney insufficiency.

Generally CAPD is used in patients older than 65 years, patients with diabetic nephropathology, children before transplantion and patients with severe cardio vascular instability or vascular access not sufficient for hemodialysis. CAPD also is preferred in the treatment of HIV infected dialysis patients.

Despite this positive experience, CAPD still is discussed controversially and applied internationally in varying intensity (UK 41 %, Canada 28 %, USA 10 %, FRG less than 5 %).

Those refusing CAPD claim the risk of peritonitis to be a strong argument against CAPD, even though the application of thorough disinfection procedures may yield peritonitis free intervals up to 22 months and even more.

Criticism comes from the fact that all presently used CAPD techniques work with a more or less open system. That means, at every exchange of a bag a tube connection has to be separated and closed, resulting in two open ends intermediate. These are exposed to the normal none-sterile environment offering colony forming units a possibility to enter.

Depending on the therapeutic demand, additional disinfection such as rinsing (e.g. y-connection or 5F-connection) UV-irradiation or thermal treatment may help to improve the hygienic situation. The training and reliability of the patient, however, will influence the hygienic quality heavily.

A potential breakthrough in the reduction of peritonitis risk may be achieved by employing an entirely new concept, the concept of closed CAPD. This concept allows for the first time in CAPD to perform the exchange of solution bags sterilely in a closed system.

The necessary sterile connecting device produced by DuPont and marketed by Gambro is a compact, portable instrument to make a sterile, welded connection between two pieces of tubing which are sterile on the inside, but maybe contaminated on the outside. A microprocessor-control system within this rechargable battery-operated unit ensures fail-safe operation for every weld (Fig. 1).

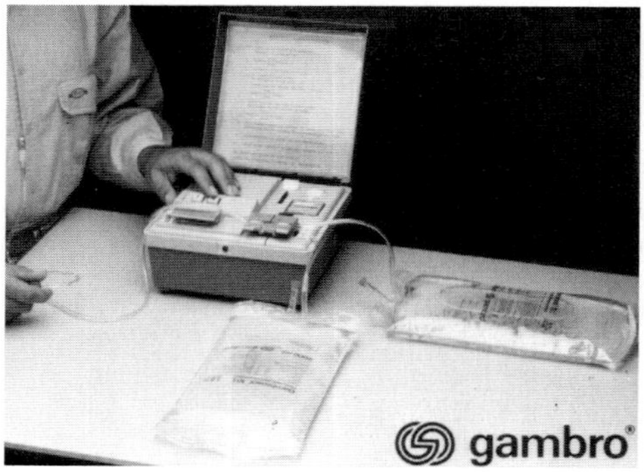

Fig. 1.

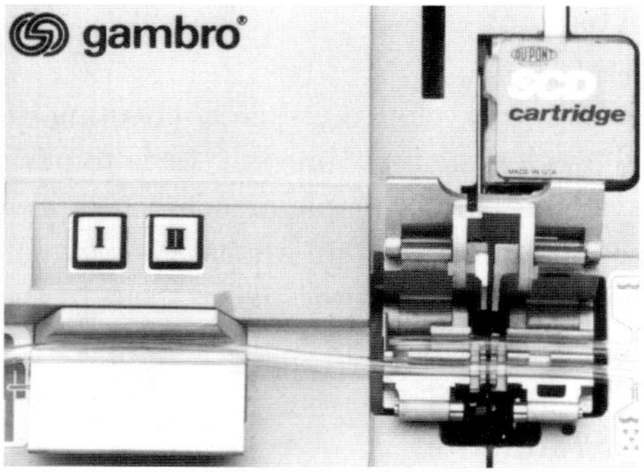

Fig. 2.

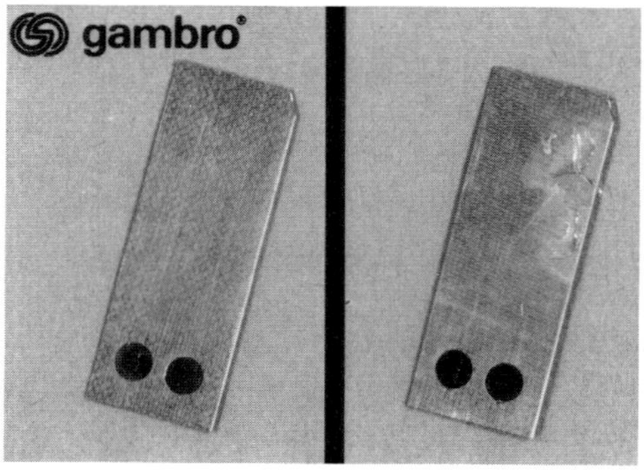

Fig. 3.

The sterile connecting device processing is an easy and simple procedure. The existing system tubing coming from the patient and going to the bag with the drained solution is placed in the front slot of the unit and the tubing with the fresh solution to be connected, is placed in the rear (Fig. 2). Then, at the push of a button, a welding wafer (Fig. 3) heats to 260° C and melts through both pieces of tubing. With the wafer still in position, the left tubing holder moves to line up with the tubing of the new bag. The device simultaneously retracts the wafer and sterilely welds the tubes together. The heated wafer continuously ensures sterility

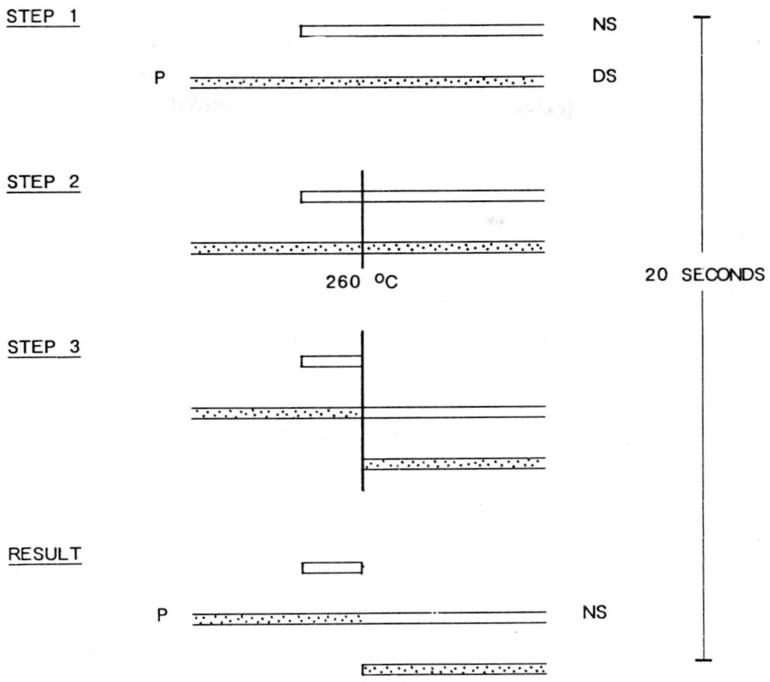

Fig. 4. Principle of SCD-closed CAPD.

of the system. A functionally closed system to external environmental contaminants is thus maintained throughout the entire process (Fig. 4).

Patients can easily be trained in this process and accept the system very well. Not only grown-ups but also children as well as blind patients have demonstrated to work successfully with the sterile connecting device.

The evaluation of the sterile connecting device was done physically, microbiologically, chemically, biologically and toxicologically. Starting with the physically evaluation tensile strength testing demonstrated tensile strength after the welding process of more than 80 % of the strength of unwelded tubing.

Particulate studies with scanning electron microscopy showed no evidence of particle generation through the welding process.

The microbiological evaluation proved sterility in several thousand welds challenged with B. circulans and Staph. epidermitis employing tubings filled with culture medium. In the chemical evaluation for liberation of volatiles, extractable solutes and trace metals sophisticated analysis methods as gas chromatography, mass spectrometry and atomic absorbtion demonstrated no release of toxic volatiles or changes in the concentration of extractables. No copper release from wafers was observed.

The biological evaluation was done by performing the welding process with tubings filled with whole blood. In all cases there was no difference versus unwelded controls regarding parameters like glucose, plasma HB, DPG, ATP, and others. (These results are the basic rationale for employing the sterile connecting device in transfusions, for which originally it was developed).

The toxicological evaluation was performed in vitro and animal toxicity studies (tissue overlay and implant) in which no difference was observed in welded versus unwelded tubings.

The reduction of peritonitis risk is documented in a number of publications. Hamilton [1] was able to demonstrate that in a group of 31 high risk patients, who had one or more episodes of peritonitis per year during a previous spike period, the frequency of peritonitis was reduced by 50 % upon employing closed CAPD. Adams and Evans [2] obtained peritonitis free intervals in a group of 14 patients of more than 21 months after employing the sterile connecting device instead of the spike system.

In summary one can conclude that sterile closed CAPD allows for sterile bag exchange. This procedure is performed very quickly within 20 seconds. Closed CAPD reduces the peritonitis risk. It is easy to handle and thus contributes favorably to reduce the training time. It can be speculated that this system will help CAPD to gain a bigger share in the treatment of dialysis patients.

References

[1] HAMILTON, R. W., et al.: Reduction in peritonitis frequency by the DuPont sterileconnection device. *TASAIO* 31: 651 (1985).

[2] ADAMS, EVANS: Proceedings of the 7th Annual CAPD Conference, Kansas City, 106-107 (1987).

First Results with the New Closed CAPD-System

U. WEBER, R. BAMBAUER

Abstract

The experience with a new closed CAPD-system is reported here. In a 49 years old female patient with end stage renal disease, this modification of CAPD with a sterile connection device was applied first in 1988.

Introduction

The modern era of clinical peritoneal dialysis started with the introduction of the continuous ambulatory peritoneal dialysis (CAPD) by Popovich et al. in 1978 [1]. As ever, peritonitis continues to be a major complication though many efforts have been made to reduce the incidence, especially by means of technical improvements.

Case Report

We report on our first experiences with the new closed CAPD-system treating a 49 years old female patient with an end stage renal disease. She considered CAPD to be the most acceptable dialysis method to exhibit normal activity in daily living

July, 7th: A Tenckhoff catheter was inserted in our Department of Surgery: afterwards the patient was trained.

Three weeks later: We saw an incomplete catheter obstruction resulting from migration towards the left hypocondrium. A Fogarty catheter was aseptically inserted and a relocation of the Tenckhoff could be achieved (in our Department of Radiodiagnostic). After further catheter dislodgments a catheter revision was necessary.

August, 17th: A catheter removal and replacement was performed. Subsequent x-rays demonstrated that the catheter was placed correctly. Further treatment was free of complications, and the patient tolerated the procedure well.

September, 8th: The patient presented the clinical signs of a peritonitis. We found Staphylococcus aureus as the infective agent, cultured from the peritoneal fluid. The therapeutic regimen included peritoneal lavage and antibiotic treatment, which was followed by a complete cure.

The contamination path was obviously a transluminal route through a leaky welding seam caused by an incompletely recharged welding device.

Discussion

Peritonitis does still represent a dangerous complication to the peritoneal dialysis patient. The contamination path includes possibilities originating in the dialysis system as well as a mode of infection originating in the patient. For example: A faulty application technique or a hematogenic dissemination. The first named possibilities can be influenced by optimization of training and technique of the system. The development of this new connector technology could be a most promising innovation.

If the reported modification of CAPD with a sterile connection device will be an alternative to reduce the incidence of peritonitis it must be proved by further investigation including a large number of patients.

References

[1] POPOVICH, R. P., J. W. MONCRIEF, K. D. NOLPH, A. J. GHODS, Z. J. TWARDOWSK: Continuous ambulatory peritoneal dialysis. *Ann. intern. Med.* 88: 449-456 (1978).

Reduced Risk for Leakage by Placing Peritoneal Dialysis Catheter through the Rectus Muscle

B. STEGMAYR, B. HEDBERG, B. SANDZEN, A. M. WIKDAHL

Abstract

Frequent postoperative leakage of peritoneal dialysis fluid occurred when we used the technique where a double cuff Tenckhoff catheter was placed in the linea alba. From October 1987 we started to insert the Tenckhoff catheter about 3 cm laterally of the linea alba. Under local anaesthesia, the anterior and posterior fascial blade of the rectus muscle were cut while the muscular part was carefully split apart. The inner Tenckhoff catheter-cuff was placed ventral to the peritoneal membrane and fixed with a purse string suture of Dexon®. The same type of suture was used to adhere the inner cuff to the inner fascial blade. The outer fascial blade was sutured similarly around the exit of the catheter with single stiches above and below. The tunnel was made in the subcutis. The patients were asked to be bedridden for three days to allow healing the wound. Operation was performed consecutively in 12 men and six women with a mean age of 53 years (range 25-81 years). Eight of them were older than 60 years. The median treatment time was four months (range 1-8 months). In no patient did leakage develop, neither in the first postoperative period nor in the follow-up course. In total three peritonitis incidences occurred during 102 months (1/34). One of them had ascites when the catheter was inserted and a mycobacteria peritonitis was diagnosed in the follow up. In three patients, there has been an exit site infection. In none of them peritonitis could be referred to invasive bacteria from the tunnel. In one case the outer cuff was loosened after mechanical trauma but no peritonitis occurred during the observation period. One patient was given initially 2 l of peritoneal dialysis fluid immediately postoperatively instead of the normally administered volume of 1.0 l.

Conclusion: The lateral insertion technique is easy, may be performed in local anesthesia and allows immediate start of the peritoneal dialysis. The use of three purse string sutures may lower risk for invasion of bacteria from outer site into the peritoneal space. In patients who start peritoneal dialysis, postoperative fluid leakage may be seen in 7-24% [1-10]. The leaks often occur early in the postoperative course [2, 7]. Leakage may be reduced if the start of peritoneal dialysis is delayed for several days after catheter insertion [11] or if the insertion in made by lateral approach [2, 6, 12-15].

We investigated the incidence of leakage and the risk for peritonitis by tunnel infections in a consecutive group of patients in whom the insertion of the catheter was performed by a modified lateral approach.

Materials and Methods

At our hospital we had an incidence of early leakage of about 20 percent by the midline insertion of Tenckhoff catheters (TeC) although the patients were bedridden for three days. This urged us to change the technique to a modified lateral insertion given below. Peritoneal dialysis (PD) was started in 18 consecutive patients, 12 men and six women, of mean age 53 years (SD $\pm$18, range 25-81 years). Eight of them were older than 60 years. All patients were treated by PD fluids from Baxter Travenol (Stockholm, Sweden). Preoperatively, all patients received 750 mg of cefuroxime and then twice a day for two days.

The TeC was inserted about 3 cm laterally of the linea alba and, in most patients, at the right side with the intraperitoneal part pointing to the left (TeC aided downwards by peristaltics of the colon). Local anaesthesia was used with all patients. The anterior fascial blade of the rectus muscle was cut while the rectus muscle was carefully split and the epigastric vessels avoided.

A purse string suture was fixed in the dorsal fascial blade prior to a small incision and a similar procedure was performed with the peritoneum. The TeC was stiffened temporarily by the use of a stylet and the intra-abdominal part was then easily directed towards the lower abdomen on the opposite side. The inner TeC-cuff was placed ventral to the peritoneal membrane and fixed with the purse string suture of Dexon®. The purse string suture in the dorsal/inner fascia of the rectus muscle was then adhered to the outer end of the inner cuff. By a third purse string suture, the outer fascial blade was fixed around the catheter extruding from the muscle. Single stitches were secured in the proximal and distal part of the fascia of the rectus muscle. A tunnel was made with the aim of obtaining the subcutaneous part of the TeC straight, thus reducing risk for extrusion of the outer cuff located 1 cm inside the skin exit of the TeC. The dialysis was started, immediately after insertion of the TeC, usually by the use of 1 l of PD fluid. In two patients, by mistake, 2 l of PD fluid were instilled i.p. during the first day.

Exchanges of PD fluid were, during the first day, given every hour in day time, up to eight times, and every second to fourth hour during the night. The extent of exchanges was successively reduced during the following days. Most patients were asked to be bedridden during the first three postoperative days to avoid distension in the operation wound. (A few patients did, however, leave their bed already a few hours after the operation.)

Results

In no patient did leakage develop, neither in the first postoperative period nor in the follow-up course. The median treatment time was four months (six, range 1-8 months). Three peritonitis incidences occurred during a total of 102 months (1/34). One of the patients had ascites when the catheter was inserted and a mycobacteria peritonitis was diagnosed in the follow up. Exit site infection developed in three patients after 4.5 and 5 months, respectively, on peritoneal dialysis. These patients were identical with those who got peritonitis. The bacteria cultured from the peritoneal dialysis fluid were not identical with strains cultured from the exit site infection. In two of them the catheter was removed and a new one was inserted on the opposite side. No deep tunnel infections were seen during the surgical removal. In the third case the outer cuff was loosened after mechanical trauma but no peritonitis occurred during the observation period. No hernia developed at the site of operation.

Discussion

The change from the midline to the lateral approach eliminated the leakage problem in our patients. By the use of a triple layer purse string suture we think that wound healing is considerably enhanced and that the dislocation of the inner cuff is greatly restricted. The operation is performed in less than 45 minutes and can easily be done under local anaesthesia, even in a high-risk patient. The possibility to start dialysis immediately after surgery is of great advantage in highly uremic patients and may also be possible in those who start peritoneal dialysis in the course of an acute renal failure. By the use of a stylet to direct the intraperitoneal placement of the TeC, almost no problems occurred with the filling and drainage and no reoperation was needed for other causes than severe peritonitis or tunnel infection. It is noteworthy that the tunnel infections in our patients never penetrated the ventral fascial blade and were only located in the outer part of the subcutaneous tunnel. By the use of the lateral approach leakage of dialysis solution was a minor problem [12] or not seen at all [15]. They used only one purse string suture and the cuff was placed within the muscle bundle. We think that the adherence of the inner cuff within the muscle bundle might cause more inconvenience for the patient than if it is placed between the peritoneal membrane and the inner fascia. This latter approach enables a good local fixation of the catheter.

With this technique we aim to shorten the time in bed from three to two days postoperatively. This technique may be partly responsible for the overall low incidence of peritoneal infections by preventing invasion of bacteria from the subcutaneous tunnel to the peritoneal space.

In conclusion, these results suggest the use of a lateral approach. The fixation of the TeC by three purse string sutures may further restrict dislocation and leakage. The technique allows immediate start of dialysis.

Acknowledgements

We thank Lena Granbom for skilful care of the patients. The study was supported by grants from Norrlands Njursjukas Förbund.

References

[1] MALLONGA, E. T., F. VAN COEVORDEN, E. W. BOESCHOTEN, J. SOUTHWOOD, R. T. KREDIET: Surgical problems in continuous ambulatory peritoneal dialysis (CAPD). *Neth. J. Surg.* 34(3): 117-122 (1982).

[2] PONCE, S. P., A. PIERRATOS, S. IZATT, R. MATHEWS, R. KHANNA, G. ZELLERMAN, D. G. OREOPOULUS: Comparison of the survival and complications of three permanent peritoneal dialysis catheters. *Peritoneal dialysis bulletin* 2: 82-86 (1982).

[3] BROWN, M. W., D. H. N. HAMILTON, B. J. R. JUNOR: Surgical complications in patients on continuous ambulatory peritoneal dialysis. *J. Roy. Coll. Surg. Edinb.* 28: 141-146 (1983).

[4] GLOOR, H. J., W. K. NICHOLS, M. I. SORKIN, B. F. PROWANT, J. M. KENNEDY, B. BAKER, K. D. NOLPH: Peritoneal access and related complications in continuous ambulatory peritoneal dialysis. *Am. J. Med.* 74: 593-598 (1983).

[5] GREFBERG, N., B. G. DANIELSON, P. NILSSON, J. WAHLBERG: Comparison of two catheters for peritoneal access in patients undergoing continuous ambulatory peritoneal dialysis (CAPD). *Scand. J. Urol. Nephrol.* 17: 343-346 (1983).

[6] OLCOTT, C., C. A. FELDMAN, N. S. COPLON, M. L. OPPENEHIMER, J. T. MEHIGAN: Continuous ambulatory peritoneal dialysis: technique of catheter insertion and management of associated surgical complications. *Am. J. Surg.* 146: 98-102 (1983).

[7] FRANCIS, D. M. A., P. K. DONNELLY, P. S. VEITCH, G. PROUD, R. M. R. TAYLOR, J. M. RAMOS, M. K. WARD, R. WILKINSON, R. W. ELLIOTT, D. N. S. KERR: Surgical aspects of continuous ambulatory peritoneal dialysis: 3 years experience. *Br. J. Surg.* 71: 225-229 (1984).

[8] BULLMASTER, J. R., S. K. MILLER, R. K. FINLEY, L. M. JONES: Surgical aspects of the Tenckhoff peritoneal dialysis catheter. A 7 year experience. *Am. J. Surg.* 149: 339-342 (1985).

[9] DI PAOLO, N., A. MANGANELLI, F. STRAPPAVECCIA, M.DE MIA, E. GAGGIOTTI: A new technique for insertion of the Teckhoff peritoneal dialysis catheter. *Nephron* 40: 485-487 (1985).

[10] FINAN, P. J., P. J. GUILLOU: Experience with surgical implantation of catheters for continuous ambulatory peritoneal dialysis. *Ann. Royal Coll. Surg. Engl.* 67: 190-192 (1985).

[11] KHANNA, R., D. G. OREOPOULUS, N. DOMBROS, S. I. VAS, P. WILLIAMS, H. E. MEEMA, H. HUSDAN, R. OGILVIE, G. ZELLERMAN, D. A. K. RONCARI, S. CLAYTON, S. IZATT: Continuous ambulatory peritoneal dialysis after 3 years: Still a promising treatment. *Peritoneal dialysis bulletin* 1: 24-34 (1981).

[12] HELFRICH, G. B., B. W. PECHAN, M. R. ALJANI, W. F. BARNARD, T. A. RAKOWSKI, J. F. WINCHESTER: Reduction of catheter complications with lateral placement. *Perit. Dial. Bull. Suppl.* 3: 2-4 (1983).

[13] VERREET, P. R., V. RÖTZSCHER, B. ULRICH: Implantationstechnique des Oreopoulos-Zellermann-Katheters zur Peritonealdialyse. *Chirurg* 54: 609-612 (1983).

[14] SPENCE, P. A., R. MATHEWS, R. KHANNA: Improved results with a paramedian technique for the insertion of peritoneal dialysis catheters. *Surg. Gyn. Obstet.* 161: 585-587 (1985).

[15] PATTERSON, R. B., T. V. WHELAN, C. W. SCHWAB: Insertion of peritoneal dialysis catheters: The lateral approach. *Southern Med. J.* 81: 577-579 (1988).

Permanent Peritoneal Catheter in Patients on CAPD

A. Bren, J. Drinovec, J. Lindič, A. Guček

Abstract

From June 1983 to June 1988 45 peritoneal catheters were implanted to 37 patients with terminal renal failure: 36 Tenckhoff catheters with two cuffs (TC2C), one Tenckhoff catheter with one cuff (TC1C), four Toronto-Western-Hospital catheters (TWHC), three Goretex catheters (GC) and one silicone catheter (SC). They were implanted with a straight medial cut with subcutaneous tunnel, only GC catheters were implanted with a direct surgical technique. Overall catheter survival was 495 months: 384 months for TC2C, 51 for TC1C, 56 for TWHC, 33 for GC and four months for SC. We have observed 19 cases of exit site infections at TC2C, one at TC1C, one at TWHC and five at GC. The tunnel tract infection was registered in two cases of TC2C, a dislocation in two cases of TC2C, an outflow obstruction in four cases of TC2C and in one case of TWHC. Catheter loss was due to recurrent peritonitis (14), drainage obstruction (2), technical impairments (3), avulsion (1), sepsis (1), abdominal hernia (1) and exitus (5). The relationship between early and late disfunction was 1 to 1.6.

Introduction

The preservation of a well-functioning access to the peritoneal cavity is the key to successful chronic peritoneal dialysis [1, 2]. Therefore a careful follow-up of catheter-related complications is needed [3].

In our overview we are discussing the causes of catheter malfunction and catheter loss in our patients with end stage renal failure treated with continuous ambulatory peritoneal dialysis (CAPD).

Patients and Methods

From June 1983 to June 1988 CAPD was performed in 37 patients (patients) (20 men, 17 women) from 25 to 77 years. 17 patients were diabetics (nine with diabetes mellitus type I, nine with type II). In four cases the cause of end stage renal failure was analgetic nephropathy, in one patient chronic pyelonephritis, in three chronic glomerulonephritis, in four patients hypertensive nephroangiosclerosis, in two patients amyloidosis and in six patients unknown nephropathy.

For performing of CAPD the Travenol system II and III, Fresenius system and peritoneal dialysis solution Peritodial® with 1.36 % of glucose and 3.86 % of glucose in solution were used.

The CAPD catheters were inserted with a straight medial cut with subcutaneous tunnel with a direct surgical technique in the case of Goretex catheter.

Exit site infection was defined by purulent drainage and/or erythema at the catheter-epidermal interface and positive culture [3, 4].

Tunnel tract infection was defined by induration of the area between the two cuffs with or without abcess formation or purulent drainage [3, 4].

Bacterial or fungal peritonitis was defined by purulent dialysis effluent, 100 or more leucocytes/ml of effluent, abdominal pain and positive culture [3-5].

Catheter outflow failure was defined by total or partial obstruction of outflow drainage requiring catheter replacement.

Catheter dislocation was assessed by the position of the catheter tip in radiographs.

Results

From June 1983 to June 1988 45 peritoneal catheters were inserted: 36 Tenckhoff's catheters with two cuffs (TC2C), one Tenckhoff's catheter with one cuff (TC1C), four Toronto-Western-Hospital catheters (TWHC), three Goretex catheters (GC) and one Silicone catheter (SC).

Overall catheter survival was 495 treatment months (11 months per patient): 384 months for TC2C (10.7 months/patients), 51 for TC1C (is still functioning), 56 months for TWHC (14 months/patients), 33 months for GC (11 months/patients) and four months for SC (removed because of exitus).

Table one shows catheter failures in regard to the type of implanted CAPD catheter.

Table 1. Causes of catheter failures.

Complication	TC2C	TC1C	TWHC	GC	SC	Total	%
Exit site infection	19	1	1	5	0	26	57.8
Tunnel tract infection	2	0	0	0	0	2	4.4
Dislocation	2	0	0	0	0	2	4.4
Outflow obstruction	4	0	1	0	0	5	11.1
Catheter loss	19	0	5	3	0	27	60.0

Outflow obstructions and technical impairments occured in the first three weeks after catheter implantation but all the other complications were observed in the late period.

The causative agents in exit site or tunnel tract infections were Staphylococcus aureus and epidermidis.

The causes of peritoneal catheter loss are presented in Table 2. The main causative microorganism of treatment resistant bacterial peritonitis was Staphylococcus saphrophyticus, rarely Acinetobacter. In the case of fungal peritonitis mostly fungi from Cephalosporium sp. were isolated.

Drainage obstruction was due to dislocation of the intraperitoneal segment of the catheter and omentum entanglement, the catheter could not be released without surgical intervention. It is not clear whether observed technical impairments (eroded cuff, leakage of external part of catheter) were present in vitro.

Table 2. Causes of peritoneal catheter loss.

Complication	TC2C	TC1C	TWHC	GC	SC	Total	%
Recurrent peritonitis							
– bacterial	7	0	1	2	0	10	22.2
– fungal	2	0	2	0	0	4	8.8
Drainage obstruction	2	0	0	0	0	2	4.4
Technical impairments	3	0	0	0	0	3	6.6
Avulsion	1	0	0	0	0	1	2.2
Sepsis	1	0	0	0	0	1	2.2
Abdominal hernia	1	0	0	0	0	1	2.2
Exitus	2	0	2	1	0	5	11.1

Avulsion is a rare complication and in our case it happened in an incooperative and depressive female patient.

In one patient observed sepsis was probably caused by Corynebacterium, isolated from the bowel and peritoneal effluent of previously asymptomatic patient.

The cause of death in seven patients was not related to the CAPD treatment procedure.

The relationship of early to late disfunctions was 1 to 1.6.

Discussion and Conclusions

Peritoneal catheter function and survival depends on the type of complications which develop after placement. In the early period (during first three weeks) catheter malfunction is mainly due to obstruction, dislodgement into upper abdomen, fibrin, blood cloths or omentum ingrowth and technical impairments [6, 7], as is confirmed in our studies too.

A permanent access to the peritoneal cavity and impairment of immune response in uremic patients treated with CAPD [8] is a risk factor for developing skin infections and peritonitis, which is the major cause of drop-out from CAPD program in our patients in the late period of treatment.

On the ground of our experience we do not favor the implantation of any used catheters. An ideal catheter is not available and all the utilized devices can present some important complications [9, 10].

References

[1] NOLPH, K. D. (ed.): Peritoneal dialysis. Martinus Njihoff Publ: Boston 1985.

[2] BREN, A.: Continuous ambulatory peritoneal dialysis. Univ. of Edvard Kardelj: Ljubljana 1985.

[3] OREOPOULUS, D. G., G. BAIRD-HEFRICH, R. KHANNA, G. M. LUM, R. MATTHEWS, K. PAULSEN, Z. J. TWARDOWSKI, S. I. VAS: Peritoneal catheters and exit-site practises: current recommendations. *Peritoneal dialysis bulletin* 3: 130-138 (1987).

[4] BUONCRISTIANI, U.: Exit site and tunnel infection, pp. 165-169. In: LA GRECA, G., S. CHIARMONTE, A. FABRIS, M. FERIANI, S. RONCO (eds.): Peritoneal dialysis. Proceedings of third international course on peritoneal dialysis. Wichtig Edit.: Milano 1988.

[5] DRINOVEC, J., A. BREN, A. GUCEK, J. LINDIC, A. KANDUS, R. PONIKVAR: The treatment of Staphylococcus peritonitis in patients continuous peritoneal dialysis. *Chemiotherapia* 7: 46-49 (1988).

[6] ALLON, M., J. M. SOUCIE, E. J. MACON: Complications with permanent peritoneal dialysis catheters: experience with 154 percutaneously placed catheters. *Nephron* 48: 8-11 (1988).

[7] SCHLEIFER, R., H. ZIEMEK, B. P. TEEHAN, M. H. SIGLER, G. S. GILGORE: Migration of peritoneal catheters: personal experience and survey of 72 other units. *Peritoneal dialysis bulletin* 3: 189-193 (1987).

[8] CAROZZI, S., M. G. NASINI, S. LAMPERI: Cellular and humoral defense mechanism in peritoneal dialysis, pp. 91-95. In: LA GRECA, G., S. CHIARMONTE, A. FABRIS, M. FERIANI, S. RONCO (eds.): Peritoneal dialysis. Proceedings of third international course on peritoneal dialysis. Wichtig Edit.: Milano 1988.

[9] BIERMAN, M. H., J. KASPERBAUER, A. KUSEK, M. D. HAMMEKE, R. J. JR. FITZGIBBONS, J. D. EGAN: Peritoneal catheter survival and complications in end stage renal disease. *Peritoneal dialysis bulletin* 4: 229-233 (1985).

[10] CHIARMONTE, S., M. FERIANI, A. FABRIS, C. RONCO, L. BRAGATINI, A. BRENDOLAN, M. MILAN, J. DELL' AQUILA, P. CONZ, G. LA GRECA: Catheter malfunction, pp. 161-163. In: LA GRECA, G., S. CHIARMONTE, A. FABRIS, M. FERIANI, S. RONCO (eds.): Peritoneal dialysis. Proceedings of third international course on peritoneal dialysis. Wichtig Edit.: Milano 1988.

Peritoneal Access: Clinical Applications

Microbial Colonization of Parenteral Nutrition Catheters. A Prospective Trial on Microbial Sources, Access Routes and Tunnellization Technique.

G. Panarello, M. De Cicco, V. Chiaradia, H. De Baz,
A. Fracasso, V. Testa, G. Santini, F. Tesio

Abstract

To evaluate whether tunnelling of polyurethane venous catheter for parenteral nutrition reduce the incidence of catheter related microbial colonization, 60 patients were randomized to traditional subclavian catheterization (group A) or to subcutaneous catheter tunnelling (group B). Microbiologic studies included saprophytic flora evaluation in patients and nurses. Furthermore, cutaneous insertion site swab, hemoculture, culture of infused solution and segments cultures (two in group A and three in group B) were performed in all patients. Intravascular segment was more frequently colonized in group A (10 vs. 2 $p = 0.02$), and bacterial migration from insertion site to intravascular segment was higher in group A (6 vs. 0 $p < 0.05$). Catheter hub contamination was responsible in six out of 12 microbial colonization cases, in four of the six positive cases the isolated bacterium was present in the nurses charged of bag change.

Tunnellization decreases microbial colonization of intravascular catheter by inhibiting microbial migration along the catheter.

Introduction

Multimodal treatment of oncological patients often requires the institution of a central venous access for parenteral nutrition (PN). Previous data indicates an incidence of central venous catheter (CVC) related sepsis during PN ranging between 6-28 % [1, 2]. Sepsis is therefore a frequent and life threatening complication of long term PN.

According to some authors the route most frequently followed by microorganisms colonizing the CVC is its cutaneous insertion [3], while other authors point at the CVC hub, contaminated by line changes as the main source of infection [1]. The role of tunnelling in the prevention of sepsis is presently controversial [2, 4, 5]. Subcutaneous tunnelling appears, however, to be ineffective when the CVC is made of materials with low biological inertness [4]. Bozzetti et al. showed that CVC microbial colonization (MC) is about five to eight times more frequent than sepsis [6]. In our institution the incidence of CVC related sepsis is 5 %, while MC is about

30 % [7]. A prospective randomized study to evaluate polyurethane (PUR) CVC related MC in oncological patients receiving PN was activated at our institution in June 1986. MC was preferred to sepsis as target of this study to cut down the size of the trial. The colonization of the intravascular, tunnelled and extracutaneous segments of the CVC and its correlation with microorganisms isolated from patients and nurses were also investigated. The results of this study are the subject of the present report.

Materials and Methods

From June 1986 to June 1987, 60 oncological patients requiring a CVC for PN were randomized to direct insertion of the CVC in the subclavian vein (group A) or to 10 cm subcutaneous tunnelling of the CVC (group B). Venous catheterization was performed in the operating theatre, under strict asepsis by one of us (M.D.C.). Only PUR CVCs were employed. Superior vena cava was reached through percutaneous puncture of the subclavian vein according to the technique described by Testart [8].

Following radiological confirmation of the correct CVC position, CVC was tunnelled, only in group B patients. In both groups 5 cm catheter was left extracutaneous and the skin fixed hub was connected to a 50 cm extension partly included in the sterile occlusive dressing of the CVC. The extension was replaced at every dressing. Dressing was performed three times per week only by specially trained nurses from the Clinical Nutrition Service wearing mask, gloves, gown and cap. Bag and infusion set changes were performed daily by nurses (not specially trained) from pertinent Clinical Division. Our patients did not carry other intravenous devices or were admitted to an intensive care unit. In all patients, CVC was only used for the infusion of the nutrient mixture which was prepared in the Pharmacy Department in a laminar flow hood in 3 l size bags.
Microbiologic procedures were as follows:

- before CVC insertion: skin, rectal and pharyngeal swabs in order to study the saprophyte patients flora;
- after CVC insertion: skin swab at CVC insertion site (3 cm diameter skin area around the puncture site) before each dressing, hemoculture and culture of the infused solution in the occurrence of sepsis;
- at CVC removal: skin swab at the insertion site, hemoculture, culture of the last infused solution, culture of 5 cm intravascular and 5 cm extracutaneous CVC segments in both groups and 5 cm tunnelled segment in group B patients.

The use of antibiotics prior to CVC removal was not allowed. Nurses doing dressing and those charged of infusion set change underwent skin and oropharyngeal swab weekly.

Skin, pharyngeal, rectal swabs and hemocultures were studied according to conventional methods for bacterial (aerobic) and fungal growth. CVC segments were studied according to a modified Georgiade method [9]: 10 ml Tryptic Soy Broth (TBS) were added in a tube to the segment; the tube was vortexed for 90 seconds to detach eventual agents adhered to the CVC. Quantitative evaluation through subcultures in blood agar by means of calibrated loop was then performed. Subsequently, TBS was incubated at 37 ° C for a maximum of five days; in case of turbidity or at the end of incubation time, subcultures were performed. All isolates were identified for species, biotype and antibiotype. CVC related sepsis was defined as a clinical septic episode for which no other cause was detected, which subsided after catheter removal and which was confirmed by the finding of the same organism at hemoculture and at culture of the intravascular segment. Microbial colonization was defined as the presence of a positive culture of the CVC intravascular segment.

Chi square statistical method was employed for analysis of data. Patients characteristics in the two groups are reported in Table 1.

Table 1. Patient characteristics.

	Group A (non-tunnelled)	Group B (tunnelled)
Age		
– median	56	55
– range	19-78	26-78
Sex		
– male	15	16
– female	15	14
Neoplastic diseases		
– lymphomas	14	9
– gastrointestinal tract	8	10
– female genital tract	6	8
– lung	–	3
– breast	2	–

Results

CVC dwelling days and the reasons for their removal are reported in Table 2. Suspected CVC related sepsis was responsible for 10 % removals; however, of the six removed catheters, only three (5 %) were responsible for the septic episodes: two in group A and one in group B. The incidence of clinical sepsis was 6.6 % in group A and 3.3 % in group B patients (not significant). Responsible organisms were Staphylococcus species, Staphylococcus epidermidis and Staphylococcus aureus respectively. The Staph. species and the Staph. epidermidis of the two patients in group A were also cultured in the swab from the respective CVC insertion sites, while the Staph. aureus isolated in one group B patient had an identical antibiotype as the isolate from the hand skin swab of the nurse in charge of bag changes. In the other three cases of sepsis, hemocultures were positive for

Escherichia coli (source not ascertained due to death within 24 hours), Candida albicans (systemic candidiasis) and unidentified Gram negative germ (subcutaneous abscess) respectively. Persistence of symptoms after CVC removal and CVC negative cultures allowed for exclusion of CVC responsibility in the genesis of sepsis in these three patients.

Table 2. Reasons for CVC removal and dwelling time.

	Group A (non-tunnelled)	Group B (tunnelled)
Reasons for CVC removal		
– end of PN	19	18
– death	6	7
– mechanical causes	1	3
– sepsis	4	2
CVC dwelling time (days)		
– total	544	542
– average	18	18
– range	4-134	5-89

Table 3. CFUs / Catheter Segment.

Group	Bacterium	E.C.	T.	I.V.	Hemoculture
B	Staph. A.	7,000	1,000,000	1,000,000	Staph. A.
B	Staph. S.	+	+	+	No Growth
A	Staph. S.	100,000		8,600	Staph. S.
A	Staph. E.	1,000,000		1,000,000	Staph. E.
A	Staph. E.	1,300		200	No Growth
A	Staph. E.	57,000		2,800	No Growth
A	Staph. E.	12,000		4,000	No Growth
A	Staph. E.	–		+	No Growth
A	Staph. A.	+		+	No Growth
A	Pseud. F.	+		+	No Growth
A	Staph. S.	+		+	No Growth
A	Staph. S.	+		+	No Growth

E.C. : Extracutaneous; T. : Tunnelled; I.V. : Intravascular

Cultural examination performed in all CVC segments have shown contamination of the intravascular segment in 12 patients (20 %) (Table 3), ten in group A and two in group B (Table 4). In nine group A and in both group B patients intravascular segment isolate was the same as in the other segments of the respective CVC. Type of organism, number of colony forming units (CFUs) for each CVC segment when intravascular segment was positive, and respective hemocultures are reported in Table 3. In three of the group A patients, in whom the number of colonies isolated from the intravascular segment was greater than 1000, no bacteremia was seen, in disagreement with the findings of Maki [10] and Cleri [11]. CVC insertion site cultures were positive at least once in 18 patients (30 %): ten in group A and eight in group B.

In six of the group A the agent isolated at the insertion site was also present in all segments of the CVC (Table 5). In 13/18 patients CVC insertion site was positive both at dressing and at CVC removal. In four CVCs (three group A, one group B) bacteria were the same as those isolated from the skin swab of the nurses charged of infusion set changes (Table 3). No relationship between CVC isolates and pharyngeal or rectal microorganisms was found in any patient. Cultures of infused solutions were invariably negative.

Table 4. Colonization of CVC Intravascular Segment ($\chi^2 = 6.56$; $p = 0.02$).

	group A (non-tunnelled)	group B (tunnelled)
	n (%)	n (%)
Yes	10 (33.3)	2 (6.7)
No	20 (66.7)	28 (93.3)

Table 5. Positive Insertion Site ($\chi^2 = 4.75$; $p < 0.05$).

	Intravenous tunnelled CVC	Intravenous non-tunnelled CVC
Positive	0	6
Negative	8	4

Discussion

Because microbial colonization is the obligatory step before CVC related sepsis, and its incidence is many times higher than sepsis, the investigation of CVC colonization reduced of many hundred patients the size of this study and increased the statistical power.

CVC related sepsis can be explained only in 10-15 % of cases by contamination of the nutrient mixture or by hematogenous seeding [5]. According to some authors [3], CVC insertion site is the most frequent route followed by contaminating bacteria. According to this view, if CVC is tunnelled, healthy subcutaneous tissue should be an efficient wall against organism migration, provided that no polyvinylchloride CVCs are used. These CVCs appear to cause the formation of a granulating tissue channel, through which microorganisms, favored by small pressure variation due to CVC movements, may colonize the intravascular CVC segment [4].

According to other authors, the contamination of the CVC hub by maneuvers related to infusion set changes is responsible for most of the CVC related sepsis and tunnelling is therefore useless [5, 12]. Our data shows that tunnellization induces a decreased microbial colonization of the intravascular CVC.

From this study, it appears that hub and insertion site contamination equally share the responsibility for microbial colonization of CVC. In fact, in six out of 12 colonized intravascular segments, the responsible agent was the same as the isolate from CVC insertion site as identified by antibiotype (all group A); therefore tunnellization dramatically decreased the rate of bacterial migration along the catheter.

In four out of the latter six cases, the number of colonies isolated in the CVC extracutaneous segment was greater than in the intravascular segment, probably because of dilution of the microbial charge during migration along the subcutaneous external CVC surface. In the remaining six patients with intravascular segment colonization, MC seems to start from the CVC hub, since the insertion site swab (and therefore external surface of the CVC extracutaneous segment) and infused solution cultures were always negative. However in four out of six cases, bacteria isolated from the intravascular segment were the same (species and antibiotype) as those found in the skin swab of nurses in charge of bag changes. In the last two cases microbial source was not identified. Only 20 % of our patients were infected, probably because of the use of (PUR) CVCs with high biological inertness and softness. The latter two factors imply a low thrombogenicity. Intra and extraluminal fibrin deposition appears in fact to favor CVC infection [12, 13, 14]. Furthermore, CVC hub may have had a lesser importance as microbial entrance route since we employed a longer extension of the CVC hub and protected the CVC extension by occlusive sterile dressing. An additional factor is probably related to the particular care in ensuring asepsis at bandage dressing.

Conclusions

1. Accurate microbiological investigation performed on patients and staff is mandatory to recognize microbial sources and catheter colonization routes.
2. Tunnellization may substantially decrease by half intravascular CVC colonization by inhibiting microbial migration along the catheter.
3. Nurses must use aseptic techniques not only for CVC dressing but also for bag and infusion set change. All these rules may reduce CVC colonization from the actual 20 % to an excellent 3 % rate; consequently the expected sepsis incidence rate should be between 0.5 and 1 %.

Acknowledgements

We gratefully thank patients, Medical, Surgical Oncology and Clinical Nutrition nurses, and principally Mrs. Anna Maria Cigana for cooperation and Miss Paola Brunetti for secretarial assistance.

References

[1] Sitges-Serra, A., J. Linares, J. L. Perez, E. Jaurrieta, L. Lorente: A randomized trial on the effect of tubing changes on hub contamination and catheter sepsis during parenteral nutrition. *JPEN* 9: 322-325 (1985).

[2] Keohane, P. P., B. J. M. Jones, H. Attril, A. Cribb, J. Northover, P. Frost, D. B. A. Silk: Effect of catheter tunnelling and a nutrition nurse on catheter sepsis during parenteral nutrition. *Lancet* 2: 1388-1390 (1983).

[3] Bjorson, H. S., R. Colley, R. H. Bower, V. P. Duty, J. T. Scwartz-Fulton, J. E. Fischer: Association between microorganism growth at the catheter insertion site and colonization of the catheter in patients receiving total parenteral nutrition. *Surgery* 92: 720-727 (1982).

[4] Von Meyenfeldt, M. M. F., J. Stapert, P. C. M. De Jong, P. B. Soeters, R. I. C. Wesdorp, J. M. Greep: TPN catheter sepsis: lack of effect of subcutaneous tunnelling of PVC catheters on sepsis rate. *JPEN* 4: 514-517 (1980).

[5] Sitges-Serra, A., J. Linares: Tunnells do not protect against venous catheter-related sepsis. *Lancet* 1: 459-460 (1984).

[6] Bozzetti, F., G. Terno, G. Bonfanti, D. Scarpa, A. Scotti, M. Ammatuna, G. Bonalumi: Prevention and treatment of central venous catheter sepsis by exchange via a guidewire. *Ann. Surg.* 198: 48-52 (1983).

[7] De Cicco, M., V. Chiaradia, A. Fracasso, R. Sigon, G. F. Santini, V. Testa: Tunnellizzazione vs non tunnellizzazione del catetere di poliuretano per npt: incidenza di sepsi, pp. 243-246. In: Crucitti, F., G. B. Doglietto, R. Bellantone, L. Sofo, L. Chiovini (eds.): Giornate di chirurgia oncologica V Convegno, Roma 1987.

[8] Testart, J.: À propos de la ponction des vènes-clavières. *Concours Med.* 91: 7949 (1969).

[9] Georgiade, N., M. Lucas, R. Georgiade: The use of a new potent topical antibacterial agent for the control of infection in the burn wound. *Plast. Reconstr. Surg.* 39: 349-356 (1967).

[10] Maki, D. G., C. E. Weise, H. W. Sarafin: A semiquantitative culture method for identifying intravenous-catheter related infection. *N. Engl. J. Med.* 296: 1305-1309 (1977).

[11] Cleri, D. J., M. L. Corrado, S. J. Selingman: Quantitative culture of intravenous catheters and other intravascular inserts. *J. Infect. Dis.* 141: 781-786 (1980).

[12] Stillman, R. M., F. Soliman, L. Garcia: Etiology of catheter associated sepsis. *Arch. Surg.* 112: 1497-1499 (1977).

[13] Hoshal, V. L., R. G. Anse, P. A. Hoskins: Fibrin sleeve formation on indwelling central venous catheters. *Arch. Surg.* 102: 353-358 (1971).

[14] Tanner, W. A., P. V. Delaney, T. P. Hennessy: The influence of heparin on intravenous infections. A prospective study. *Br. J. Surg.* 67: 311-312 (1980).

Intraperitoneal Cytostatic Therapy by Means of an Implantable Catheter System

P. BRANDNER, K. J. NEIS, G. BASTERT, W. SCHMIDT

Abstract

During 18 months 15 women had intraperitoneal cytostatic therapy at our department. All patients suffered from ovarian cancer of the primary stage FIGO II or III and had undergone surgery and systemic chemotherapy previously. A catheter (Port-a-Cath) was implanted on the occasion of second- or third-look-laparotomy, which was performed in order to check on the results of the foregoing therapy as well as to do a further tumor-reduction if necessary. In all patients three cycles of intraperitoneal chemotherapy were administered on the average. Some of the patients suffered from considerable discomfort. However, the rate of secondary effects was distinctly lower than in patients with systemic chemotherapy.

Although convincing success was only achieved in women who were free of tumor already pretherapeutically, we believe a large, prospective, multicentric, randomized study to be necessary in order to check on the value of intraperitoneal chemotherapy of ovarian cancer.

Introduction

The ovarian carcinoma and its metastases are confined to the intraperitoneal space in most cases. Thus, the prognosis of the patient largely depends on local progress within the abdominal cavity. This is the reason, why the local, intraperitoneal application of cytostatic drugs may become a helpful complement in the therapeutic management of ovarian carcinoma. Rather than puncturing the abdomen for every therapeutic cycle, it seems to be reasonable, to use implantable catheter systems in order to have a comfortable and save access to the peritoneal cavity.

Patients and Methods

Between February of 1987 and July of 1988 15 women had intraperitoneal cytostatic therapy at the Gynecological Department of the University Clinics Homburg/Saar, West Germany. All patients suffered from ovarian cancer of the primary stage FIGO II or III and had undergone surgery and systemic chemotherapy previously. An intraperitoneal catheter was implanted on the occasion of second- or third-look-laparotomy, which was performed in order to check on the results of the foregoing therapy, as well as to do a further tumor-reduction if necessary. As catheter we used the system Port-a-Cath, manufactured by Pharmacia, Freiburg, FRG. After removing the Dacron-muff close to the catheter's end, the silicone tube with multiple perforations was placed free into the peritoneal space close to the Douglas. Then it was plunged through the fascial planes and was tunneled subcutaneously to the lower ribs, where the port was implanted.

The intraperitoneal chemotherapy was administered in cycles of 28 days. After puncturing the port's membrane with a Huber-needle, 1.5 liters of sodium chloride 0.9 % were injected as artificial ascites in order to confirm the cytostatic's distribution in the peritoneal cavity. If necessary, antiemetics were administered as well as tranquilizers and weak analgetics. The catheter system was perfused before every cycle with 25,000 IU of heparin diluted in 10 ml of sodium chloride 0.9 %.

Results

Between February of 1987 and July of 1988, 15 patients were treated with 43 cycles of intraperitoneal cytostatic therapy. With an average of three cycles for each patient, the number of applications ranged from one up to six cycles. 20 mg of Mitoxantrone were administered in 40 cycles, three times 100 to 120 mg of Cisplatin were injected.

Patients were divided into three groups: The first group (n = 4) showed at the time of surgery and catheter implantation remaining tumor-masses exceeding two centimeters of diameter. The second group (n = 7) had tumor-residues smaller than two centimeters or even residues, which were proven only microscopically. The third group (n = 4) showed no evidence of disease at the beginning of intraperitoneal therapy.

For the four patients with tumor-residues of at least two centimeters in diameter the indication for the intraperitoneal chemotherapy was the raise of tumor-markers and progress of tumor under ongoing systemic chemotherapy or the refusal of further systemic chemotherapy by the patient. In this group, success was achieved neither clinically nor according to the tumor-markers. Intraperitoneal therapy was changed to radiation or hormonal treatment in all four cases due to tumor-progress after two cycles in average with a range from one to three cycles.

At the time of Port-a-Cath-implantation, seven patients had minimal residues of ovarian carcinoma. Two patients can not be used for a follow-up, because one of them refused therapy after two i.p.-cycles and the second one had a perforation of the port through the skin after one cytostatic cycle with consecutive explantation of the system and change to radiation therapy. On the average, the remaining five patients obtained four cycles of intraperitoneal therapy, ranging from three up to six cycles. In four cases of five a rapid tumor-progress was observed after a period of about three months, causing either the patient's death or a change in therapy. We have to emphasize, that tumor-progress in three cases of four was observed not within the abdominal cavity, but extraperitoneally in terms of retroperitoneal lymphomas or malignant pleural effusions. One woman is free of relapse having absolved four cycles of intraperitoneal chemotherapy in a period of six months.

Four patients with no evidence of disease obtained on the average three therapeutic cycles, ranging from two up to four cycles. After a period of six, seven and ten months in two cases, all patients are free of relapse clinically as well as in apparative examinations.

Severe side effects during therapy were hardly seen. One patient suffered from fever up to 38.6 degrees Centigrade in every cycle, showing no other side effects. Alopecia of the World-Health-Organisation's degree one to two was observed twice. Three patients suffered from considerable abdominal pain, being caused in one case most probably by a lacking distribution of the fluid due to intraabdominal compartments. In almost all of the cases the cytostatics and the pressure of the artificial ascites caused a sensation of nausea and abdominal discomfort, being accompanied by vomiting several times or by diarrhea. However, the smaller amount of side-effects compared to systemic, intravenuous chemotherapy was pointed out by the majority of the patients.

One patient suffered from a dislocation of the port through the skin due to an atrophia of the tissue caused by the port's pressure. There were no wound-healing problems after removing the system. The 14 remaining catheters showed no tendency to perforation. Peritonitis or an infection of the catheter was not observed in any of the patients. However, problems were seen twice when the catheter was to be taken out by retraction in local anesthesia. In both cases it had been missed to remove the Dacron-muff from the catheter causing severe intraperitoneal adhesions. Laparotomy and adhesiolysis had to be performed in order to retrieve the system.

Discussion

In most of the cases ovarian cancer is confined to the abdominal cavity [1, 2]. This fact gave rise to several studies of intraperitoneal therapy. As cytostatic drugs – single or in combination – Melphalane, 5-fluorouracil, Mitomycin C, Cisplatin, Carboplatin, Cytarabine, Mitoxantrone and others have been used [3]. In other studies immune response modifiers such as Alfa-2B-Interferon were administered intraperitoneally [4].

In the underlying study, Mitoxantrone was used in 40 out of 43 cycles due to its presumed high cytostatic activity in intraperitoneal treatment of ovarian carcinoma [5]. However, i.p.-therapy was without any benefit for patients with considerable tumor-residues. In five patients with minimal residues progress of cancer was observed four times. Good results were achieved only in the collective with no evidence of disease, so that intraperitoneal chemotherapy should be offered only to these patients. Concern should be given to extraperitoneal progress of disease in terms of lymphomas, malignant pleural effusions or other metastases under ongoing local therapy.

The unexpected bad results of the underlying study – especially in the collective with minimal residues – may be caused by the smallness of the collective and by the rather low dose of 20 mg Mitoxantrone per cycle, which is only two thirds of the dose recommended by other authors [6, 7].

Having used the Verres-needle under x-ray control before, the intraperitoneal catheter proved to be a save and comfortable access to the peritoneal cavity. In the underlying study the completely implantable catheter system Port-a-Cath was used [8]. Complications were very rare: Peritonitis or infections of the implantation site were not seen. The dislocation of the system's port, which was observed in one case, was due to atrophia of the covering skin; a local infection in that area was secondary and did not penetrate through the peritoneum. In two cases the withdrawal of the catheter in local anesthesia was not possible, because it had been missed to remove the catheter's Dacron-muff before implantation. The catheters had to be retrieved by laparotomy. Our suggestion is, always to remove the Dacron-muff in order to avoid adhesions or, even better, to convince the manufacturer, to produce the catheter without the muff. As we hear from other work-groups, non-removable catheters were left within the abdominal cavity and only the subcutaneous port was explanted; no complications were reported about.

In summary it may be stated, that we have a very satisfying access to the abdominal cavity by using implantable catheter systems with subcutaneous ports. The intraperitoneal chemotherapy of the ovarian cancer, however, has to be thought about in terms of the group of patients, who benefit from this therapy as well as in terms of the administered dose of drugs.

References

[1] COLLINS, J. M.: Pharmacokinetik rationale for drug delivery. *J. Clin. Oncol.* 2: 498-504 (1984).

[2] DEDRICK, R. L.: Theoretical and experimental bases of intraperitoneal chemotherapy. *Semin. Oncol.* 12(3), Suppl. 4: 1-6 (1985).

[3] MARKMANN, M.: Intraperitoneal antineoplastic agents for tumors principally confined to the peritoneal cavity. *Cancer Treatment Reviews* 13: 219-242 (1986).

[4] BEZWODA, W. R., J. FORDER: Intraperitoneal administration of recombinant Alfa-2B-Interferon for treatment of the ovarian carcinoma: Correlation with clonogenic stem cell assays. *Proc. ASCO* 7: 140 (1988).

[5] ALBERTS, D. S., L. YOUNG, N. MASON, S. E. SALMON: In vitro evaluation of anticancer drugs against ovarian cancer at concentrations achievable by intraperitoneal administration. *Semin. Oncol.* 12(3) Suppl. 4: 38-42 (1985).

[6] BLÖCHL-DAUM, B., H. G. EICHLER, H. RAINER, R. JAKESZ, H. SALZER, G. STEGER, J. SCHÜLLER, E. GÜNTHER, P. PROKSCH, G. EHNINGER: Phase I-study of intraperitoneal Mitoxantrone – clinical and pharmacokinetic evaluation. *Onkologie* 10(1): 54-56 (1987).

[7] ALBERTS, D. S., E. SURWIT, Y. M. PENG, T. MCCLOSKEY, V. GRAHAM, L. MCDONALD, D. ROE: Phase I-II and pharmacokinetic study of Mitoxantrone by intraperitoneal administration. *Proc. ASCO* 6: 118 (1987).

[8] PFEIFLE, C. E., S. B. HOWELL, M. MARKMAN, W. E. LUCAS: Totally implantable system for peritoneal access. *J. Clin. Oncol.* 2: 1277-1280 (1984).

Therapeutic Plasma Exchange

New Trends of Therapeutic Plasmapheresis

S. NAGANUMA, P. S. MALCHESKY, K. SAWADA, Y. NOSÉ

Abstract

In the early 1980's therapeutic plasmapheresis was projected to represent the new wave of artificial organ technologies for blood detoxication. Today, plasmapheresis technology offers an acceptable treatment modality, and is emerging as a tool for the elucidation of many kinds of disease processes. Despite the successes so far obtained with plasmapheresis, many aspects of this therapy remain to be reconsidered.

Therapeutic plasma exchange, removal of plasma from the blood and substitution of appropriate fluids for the plasma removed, has been used to treat numerous diseases, and has been the focus of the application of plasmapheresis technology. Although favorable responses to plasmapheresis were observed in some diseases, the efficacy of plasmapheresis remains unproven in a number of conditions that might be expected to respond on theoretical grounds. Besides considering the relative safety and high cost, the rationale to use plasmapheresis should be reviewed strictly now from the clinical benefit point of view.

In attempts to develop a modality for removing pathogenic macromolecules, the pioneers of this field started with whole blood exchange transfusions and then progressed to simple plasma exchange. Presently numerous studies are now ongoing on selective removal by way of on-line plasma fractionation. An aim of plasmapheresis is selective removal of pathogenic macromolecules with modification of metabolic and immunologic status of patients in an effort that end-stage patients be reduced to below the current levels.

Indication and limitation of therapeutic plasmapheresis

Plasmapheresis has expanded to the treatment of many diseases in this decade. More than one hundred diseases, for with conventional therapies are often ineffective, slow-acting, or unacceptably toxic, had been treated by plasmapheresis and its modified technologies [1], and several hundred scientific articles are being generated each year about this subject.

While the number of this disease states approved for the use of apheresis in the United States remains small due to the lack of well-defined control trials and limited reimbursement, the potential patient population that can be helped with plasma exchange and plasma treatment procedures is growing. Reportedly nearly

300,000 therapeutic plasma exchange procedures are performed annually in the United States [2].

Various methods of plasmapheresis are currently available: plasma exchange by centrifugal separation or membrane separation, and on-line plasma fractionation. The choice of method is highly dependent on the solutes to be removed and their properties. The association of biochemical or cellular abnormalities in various disease states provides the rationale for the application of plasmapheresis technologies. The assumed or actual accumulation of abnormal macromolecules in disease states suggests that their removal will correct the clinical abnormality. The primary objective in performing plasmapheresis is to remove large molecular weight solutes or protein-bound solutes. For plasmapheresis technologies to be effective, the solutes must be accessible through the circulation and exhibit favorable kinetics with respect to their rates of production and intra-tissue transfer to the plasma compartment.

Macromolecule kinetics in the body are not still well understood in many diseases. Certainly, abnormally increased levels of macromolecules and cells represent immunological and metabolic responses in the body. In diseases in which pathogenic mechanisms are known, the rational of plasmapheresis is to remove the pathogenic material from the circulation. Plasmapheresis is one method to remove macromolecules directly from the body. However, in many of the disorders in which this therapeutic procedure has been employed, it is difficult to demonstrate the presence of pathogenic substances in the plasma removed or to find a strong correlation between the amount of substance removed from plasma and clinical improvement. Thus, conclusive criteria for selecting patients who may benefit from plasmapheresis, and reliable parameters by which to judge the effectiveness of this treatment are difficult to draw, owing to the wide variability of the nature, clinical symptoms and course of the diseases [3]. The attractions of a therapeutic modality considered to be safe [4], potentially targeted at the pathogenic processes, and rapidly effective are obvious. However, there is controversy as to whether plasmapheresis alters the course of the disease state or whether there are other underlying interactions which determine the handling of macromolecules.

Since the initiation of plasmapheresis and pilot studies have begun, numerous reports of uncontrolled series and case reports of patients treated with a variety of protocols claimed effectiveness, but the degree of the effectiveness is controversial in some diseases, such as scleroderma, polymyositis, and multiple sclerosis, in which the rationale is not clear as to what the pathogenic materials are that are to be removed from the circulation [5]. The clinical approach in evaluating the effects of plasmapheresis through blinded, controlled trials has been tried on severals disease states in different fashion [1, 6-9]. However, based upon the experience of the controlled trials undertaken to date, certain limitations may be noted. The number of controlled clinical trial are still lacking in most instances to prove the efficacy of plasmapheresis. Controlled trials generally require years to complete are costly. They tend to be narrow in protocol design either through patient population selection, procedural, methodology choices and ethical problems. Further, the trials may be undertaken prior to therapy optimization, independent of the protocol design, the failure of the technology and statistical difficulties of trial design. Completion of one trial is usually followed by the design of a new trial with specification or control of a parameter initially uncontrolled. The statistical difficulties lie in the fact that we have to treat diseases that show a wide variability of its course and are present in various stages. Further, patient clinical conditions are so fluctuating as to make it difficult to allocate them to statistically comparable groups [3].

Diseases for the use of plasmapheresis as determined by their eligibility for reimbursement under Medicare [1] are limited only to several diseases, such as hyperviscosity syndrome, Goodpasture's syndrome, thrombotic thrombocytopenic purpura, myasthenia gravis, Waldenstrom's macroglobulinemia, hyperglobulinemia, rheumatoid vasculitis, pruritis of cholestatic liver disease, chronic relapsing polyneuropathy, scleroderma and polymyositis. Presently controlled trials are now neither completed nor under way for most of the common disease entities or various technologies are used in different disease stages with different treatment protocols designs. There is no satisfactory protocol and little consistency about the extent of plasmapheresis; exchange volumes may vary from minimal to extensive, there are variations in the type of replacement fluid (albumin, fresh frozen plasma, or purified protein solutions), the rate and frequency of exchange, and differences in therapeutic applications and procedures [10].

Table 1. Therapeutic plasmapheresis in the Cleveland Clinic, 1984-1988.

Therapeutics	# / Year				
	1984	1985	1986	1987	1988
Plasma Exchange	301	481	477	670	544
Cryofiltration	46	83	155	132	39
Thermofiltration	–	–	–	50	5
Lymphoplasmapheresis	36	79	21	65	91
Plateletpheresis	7	77	12	3	5
RBC collection	–	–	9	4	3
WBC collection	–	–	9	1	–
Adsorbent	–	–	2	2	–
Total procedure #	390	720	685	927	687

Simple plasma exchange

Historically, the largest data base exists for treatments by simple plasma exchange. Plasma exchange is procedually simple and can be carried out in larger hospitals and blood bank centers. At present, comparative data about more selective technologies, kinetics of macromolecules and diseases pathogenesis are limited.

Therefore, from consideration of the mechanics of operation, knowledge of therapy requirements, and available data base, simple plasma exchange is typically the treatment of choice in indicated disease states (Table 1). However, despite its extensive use, simple plasma exchange has the following disadvantage: (1) the requirement for plasma products for volume replacement; (2) the potential hyperallergic reaction or contamination (ie. virus) caused by plasma product infusion; and (3) the loss of essential plasma components.

Various biochemical and immunological deficiencies occur after frequent (ex. more than once per week) multiple plasma exchanges [11]. Thus, simple plasma exchange cannot be applied as intensively and frequently as the disease treatment may require. The ideal method of plasma treatment is that which can be performed as extensively and intensively as may be needed to correct the disease state. In addition, the supply of replacement plasma and albumin solution is limited worldwide. In 1981, over six million liters of plasma were collected in the United States in order to supply an international marketplace. That demand grew to twelve million liters in 1986. Concern about AIDS transmission through U.S.-derived plasma products has caused increased need for industry-government discussions about product safety, with requests for scientific and clinical support or verification. These concerns are continuing to cause temporary plasma product import restraints or delays [12].

Simple plasma exchange can be carried out using the various centrifugation devices or membrane technology. Membrane technology, which has advanced rapidly in the past decade, has provided an alternative to centrifugal techniques. Simple blood separation filters, introduced in the last ten years, are now available for the separation of plasma from the whole blood. Plasma separation with hollow fibers can be seen to have made adequate progress: priming volumes are smaller as a result of the reduced surface areas of today's high capacity plasma separators and plasma protein sieving coefficients are satisfactory (Table 2).

On-line Plasma Membrane Fractionation

Plasmapheresis by simple plasma exchange has several technical and clinical limitations due to the nonselective removal of plasma factors. Plasma fractionation techniques provide an alternative to simple plasma exchange and for some disease states may be preferred because of their selectively targeted removal of pathogenesis factor.

On-line plasmapheresis is defined as a treatment modality consisting of the removal of the whole blood from the patient, separation of plasma from the cellular blood components, subjecting the separated plasma to specific procedures, like membrane fractionation, or perfusion through columns with adsorbents or other fractionation processes, and the subsequent reunion of the treated plasma with the

Table 2. Physical Characteristics of Membrane Filters in Plasmapheresis (a. Plasma Separator).

Supplier or Manufacturer	Filters, Plasma separator	Membrane Material F: Hollow fiber P: Plate or pile C: Cryofiltration use	Surface Area (m^2)	Max Pore Size (μm)	Inner Fiber Diameter or Plate Spacing (μm)	Priming Volume (ml) Inner/ Outer	Number of Fibers or Plates	Length (cm) Full/ Effective	Sterilization
Travenol Lab, USA	CPS-10	Polypropylene (F)	0.17	0.55	320	17/178	800	26.0/21.4	EOG
AB Gambro, USA	Fiber plasmafilter PP	Polypropylene (F)	0.38	0.5	330	36/88	2000	21.0/17.0	*
	Fiber plasmafilter PC-1000	Polycarbonate (F)	0.27	*	270	24/*	2000	21.0/17.0	*
Cobe Lab, USA	TPE plasma separator	Polyvinylchloride (P)	0.13	0.6	*	18/*	6	22.0/16.0	EOG
Fresenius MTS, FRG	Plasmaflux P2	Polypropylene (F)	0.50	0.5	330	48/290	2250	25.0/20.0	EOG
Dideco SpA, Italy	Hemaplex BT900	Polypropylene (F)	0.20	0.5	320	18/*	900	25.4/21.0	*
Asahi Med., Japan	Plasmaflo AP-06-M	Cellulose diacetate (F,C)	0.65	0.2	370	95/*	3100	28.3/18.3	EOG
	Plasmaflo AP-03-H	Cellulose diacetate (F)	0.30	0.2	330	45/*	*	*/13.0	EOG
	Plasmaflo AP-05-H	Cellulose diacetate (F)	0.50	0.2	330	65/*	3000	26.5/15.7	EOG
	Plasmaflo AP-08-H	Cellulose diacetate (F)	0.80	0.2	330	90/*	*	*/18.3	EOG
Kuraray Co., Japan	Plasmacure type 'M'	Polyvinylalcohol (F)	0.30	0.2	300	40/*	1750	18/16	SAC
(Kawasumi Lab, Jap.)	Plasmacure type 'L'	Polyvinylalcohol (F)	0.50	0.2	300	60/*	2850	23.4/20	SAC
Toray Ind., Japan	Plasmax PS-05	Polymethylmethacrylate (F)	0.50	0.5	370	59/102	2500	22.0/17.5	r
	Plasmax PS-02	Polymethylmethacrylate (F)	0.15	*	370	19/*	960	18.0/13.5	r
Teijin, Japan	Plasma separator TP 50	Polymer alloy (F)	0.40	0.2	320	32/*	1600	*/25.0	EOG
Mitsubishi, Japan	Plasma sep. MPS 0250	Polyethylene (F)	0.50	*	270	45/*	3640	21.5/16.5	EOG
Terumo, Japan	PS-4000	Cellulose acetate (P)	0.50	0.45	80	80/120	30	45	EOG
Organon Tekn., USA	Curesis	Polypropylene (F)	0.12	0.65	330	12/*	800	25.0/*	*
Cordis Dow Inc.	Plasmafilter	Polyethylene (F)	0.70	*	270	66/*	5500	21.0/16.0	*
Nipro, Japan	Plasma separator PEX-50	Cellulose triacetate (F)	0.50	0.4	285	*/*	*	*	EOG
Kawasumi Lab, Japan	Plasma separator KPS02	Polypropylene (F)	0.20	0.6	330	23/*	*	*	SAC
	Plasma separator KPS03	Polypropylene (F)	0.30	0.6	330	34/*	*	*	SAC
	Plasma separator KPS04	Polypropylene (F)	0.40	0.6	330	46/*	*	*	SAC

EOG: Ethylene oxide gas; SAC: Steam autoclave; r: Gamma rays; *: Data not available from company.

cellular blood components and its return to the patient [10]. The general features of such systems are that they eliminate the requirement for plasma replacement products, spare the significant loss of normal plasma constituents, are constructed of well-characterized materials that may make their clinical use more easily qualified through governmental regulating agencies, and are of a design that may be less costly in production.

Membrane fractionation is the technique of passing the plasma through single or multiple filters following its separation from the blood. The principle of solute removal from plasma by membrane filtration is based on solute size exclusion. If certain macromolecules should be removed, cascade filtration (double filtration) is aimed to semiselectively removing molecules of a few million daltons molecular weight (e.g., immune complexes), a few hundred thousand daltons molecular weight (e.g., gamma globulin fractions), or below 100,000 daltons molecular weight (e.g., albumin fractions). Aiming for separation of this various types of macromolecules, several industrial firms have developed macromolecule filters of various porosities over the last decade (Table 3). However, the membranes which are available at present do not provide a good enough separation of IgG from albumin, an important objective in the treatment of most autoimmune diseases. It is possible only to separate molecules the sizes of IgM from proteins of less than 500,000 daltons in molecular weight. The efficacy of cascade filtration is highly dependent upon the selection of the membrane, the choice of macromolecules to be removed, and the operation condition. The importance of temperature conditions on solute fractionation should be particularly stressed in the process of membrane filtration as it is the most easily controlled physical parameter.

Membrane filtration techniques can be classified according to the temperature range employed since it has been shown that temperature effects the solute solute removal selectivity [11]. Cryofiltration was developed to overcome some of the disadvantages of plasma exchange. The presence of cryoglobulines and other cold aggregatable solutes in a number of disease states provided the initial rationale for the use of this method. In this procedure, the separation and cooling of plasma (above the freezing temperature, usually 4-5° C) and secondary filtration semiselectively removes the pathological macromolecules due to molecular sizes in the form of cryogel. Realizing that cryoprotein is a very often present in the autoimmune disease and infectious disease state [13], cryofiltration utilizes the phenomenon of cold separation to accelerate the effective separation of cryoprecipitable proteins, in which pathogenic molecules, such as immune complexes and antibodies, also are present. The technique of cryofiltration has been used clinically for the past nine years in the treatment of patients with rheumatoid arthritis (RA) [14], rheumatoid vasculitis [15], and cryoglobulinemias [16]. While studies in rheumatoid arthritis have been uncontrolled, these data provided the supporting evidence needed to plan the present two center double blind controlled trial that is currently underway. It is recognized that several

Table 3. Physical Characteristics of Membrane Filters in Plasmapheresis (b. Plasma Fractionator).

Supplier or Manufacturer	Filters, Second Filter	Membrane Material F: Hollow fiber T: Thermofiltration use	Surface Area (m^2)	Max Pore Size (μm)	Inner Fiber Diameter or Plate Spacing (μm)	Priming Volume (ml) Inner/Outer	Number of Fibers or Plates	Length (cm) Full/Effective	Sterilization
Dideco SpA, Italy	Albusave BT 902	Cellulose diacetate (F)	1.00	0.02	350	170/*	*	*/23.5	EOG
Enka AG	PF prototype	Cellulose acetate (F)	1.00	*	440	121/*	3000	26.5/21.5	*
Asahi Med., Japan	Cascadeflo AC-1730	Cellulose diacetate (F)	1.70	*	220	130/*	*	28.3/18.3	EOG
	Cascadeflo AC-1760	Cellulose diacetate (F)	1.70	*	220	130/*	*	28.3/18.3	EOG
	Cascadeflo AC-1770	Cellulose diacetate (F)	1.70	*	220	130/*	*	28.3/18.3	EOG
Kuraray Co., Japan	Eval filter type '2A'	Ethylenevinylalcohol (F)	1.00	0.01	200	100 ($1m^2$)	8000	23/19.0 ($1m^2$)	EOG
	Eval filter type '3A'	Ethylenevinylalcohol (F)	&	0.02	200	&	&	&	EOG
	Eval filter type '4A'	Ethylenevinylalcohol (F,T)	2.00	0.03	200	130 ($2m^2$)	11000	27/23.0 ($2m^2$)	EOG
Toray Ind., Japan	Plasmax AS-08	Polymethylmethacrylate (F)	0.80	*	370	97/156	3950	23.0/19.5	r
	Plasmax ASC-08	Polymethylmethacrylate (F)	0.80	*	370	97/156	3950	23.0/19.5	r
Teijin, Japan	TA-100	Cellulose diacetate (F)	0.80	*	250	50/*	*	*/25.0	*
	TA-200	Cellulose diacetate (F)	0.80	*	250	50/*	*	*/25.0	*
Terumo, Japan	CF-01	Cellulose acetate (F)	1.00	*	*	*/*	*	*/70	EOG

EOG: Ethylene oxide gas; r: Gamma rays; *: Data not available from company.

controlled trials [18, 19] have reported no statistically significant clinical effects using plasma exchange in the treatment of RA. Plasma exchange used in these trials differs in several respects from the on-line therapeutic process of cryofiltration. The trials utilizing plasma exchange were of relatively short duration, and fairly small volumes were treated, replacement of plasma product was required (not required in cryofiltration), and the procedures were performed using centrifugal plasma separators with citrate anticoagulation (membrane separators with heparin are used in cryofiltration). Since the first clinical use of cryofiltration over nine years ago [17], significant efforts have been devoted to understanding the phenomena associated with macromolecule removal and in extending the clinical experience. Three areas of investigation requiring attention in cryofiltration technology are clinical controlled trials, improved cryofilter designs and operation design, and patient selection.

The only available FDA approved cryofilter AP 06M is not suited to process large volumes of cryoprecipitable concentrated plasma. In clinical use this filter quickly plugs with an increased loss of albumin and globulin, and filter backwashing or replacement is required to reach the designed treatment plasma volumes. Due to these limitations, a high capacity filter was designed and now is being tried clinically in our group.

Atherosclerosis-induced coronary heart disease remains the major cause of death in developed countries [20]. It is beneficial if low density lipoprotein (LDL) is selectively removed. However, simple plasma exchange also removes high density lipoprotein (HDL), which is believed to be an antiatherogenic lipoprotein. Thus, plasmapheresis by the double filtration, thermofiltration or an LDL binding sorbent has been in the process of development for selective removal of apoprotein B containing lipoproteins. Thermofiltration is defined as on-line membrane filtration near or slightly above physiologic temperature, and is most commonly performed in the range, 35 to 42° C. One effective application of thermofiltration is the selective removal of low-density lipoproteins (LDL). The difference in molecular sizes between high-density lipoprotein (HDL) and low-density lipoproteins is about twofold. At temperatures between 37 to 45° C the sieving coefficients of LDL and total cholesterol are below 0.1 and higher plasma volumes are processable than at ambient or below temperatures. Thus, effectively all the low-density lipoproteins can be removed from the plasma with a high return of the HDL. No replacement solutions are required [10]. Most LDL-apheresis studies have been largely anecdotal. Well-designed controlled clinical studies are crucial to the assessment of LDL-apheresis as a viable medical procedure in the treatment for hypercholesterolemia induced atherosclerosis from the clinical benefit point of view [20].

Adsorption Therapy

Over the past two decades, the development and use of sorbents for drug detoxication, uremia, liver insufficiency, autoimmune disorders and familial hypercholesterolemia has escalated. Adsorbents may be defined as materials capable of binding substances in biological fliuds particularly from blood and plasma [21]. Solute removal by plasma sorption consists of plasma separation and perfusion of the plasma through a cartridge containing a sorbent. After passing through the sorbent, the treated plasma is combined with the blood cells and reinfused into the patients.

Table 4. Affinity-Type Sorbents.

Ligand or material of adsorption	Agent sorbed
Polylysin methylated	T_4 phage DNA
albumin	DNA
Anion exchange resin	
Polyanion	Bilirubin[a]
Dextran sulfate	LDL[a]
Heparin: Heparin agarose	LDL
Tryptophan IM-TR	Anti-acetycholine receptor Ab[a], IC, RF[a]
Phenylalanine IM-PH	Anti-MBP, Ab[a], IC, RF
Modified PVA gel I-02	RF, IC, Anti-DNA, Ab, Anti-RNP Ab, Anti-SM Ab
Oligosaccharide	Anti-blood type AB
Charcoal sorbent	Bilirubin, creatinine, urea, potassium
DNA	Anti-DNA Ab[a]
Ag Blood-type Ag	Anti-blood type Ab[a]
Insulin	Anti-insulin Ab
Factor VIII	Anti-Factor VIII Ab[a]
Factor IX	Anti-Factor FIX ab[a]
Anti-LDL Ab	LDL[a]
Ab Anti-α Feto Ab	α-Feto protein
Anti-HBs Ab	HBs
Anti-IgE Ab	IgE
Clq	Immune complex
Protein A	IC, IgG[a], C_3

[a]: Clinical application stage; PVA: polyvinyl alcohol; RF: Rheumatoid factor; IC: Immune complexes.

For treatment of various diseases, not only have activated charcoal and anion resins, which are general nonselective adsorbents, been used to treat liver failure and drug intoxication, but also several relatively selective adsorbents have been developed. Selective adsorption is based on chemical affinity, such as antigen antibody interaction, enzyme substrate interaction and receptor anti-receptor interaction. The types of sorbents are divided into two groups according to the principles of adsorption: nonimmunoselective (physicochemical interaction) or immunoselective (biological similarity) (Table 4). Nonimmunoselective sorbents include such general sorbents as activated charcoal, resins, and carriers with physicochemical interactions, such as the amino acid-bound resins. Immunoselective sorbents are carriers to which specific proteins have been attached. This latter category is more specific than the former, but in other aspects, such as capacity, safety and handling and storage of columns, the former group is superior to the latter [22].

In the area of sorbent technology, optimization of the process is particularly important because of the high costs of materials (such as monoclonal antibodies), presently low product demand, and the extensive studies for governmental approval.

Biomodulation effects in plasmapheresis

While plasmapheresis precedures are designed for solute removal, therapy will be influenced by the humoral and cellular modulation that will occur as a result of the treatment modality. Extracorporeal biomodulation refers to the act of effecting changes either procedully induced or procedurally associated in the cellular or biochemical milieu of the body. Since apheresis technologies effect such rapid changes in the humoral and cellular systems, the biomodulation effects should be considered in addition to the removal objectives of the procedures. Also, because of the low generation rates of the various plasma solutes and cells, the impact of such procedures will countinue beyond the apheresis procedure time.

The biocompatibility of the materials of blood and plasma contact affect the activation of complement in other blood systems, e.g. coagulation, fibrinolysis as well as effects on specific blood cells [26]. The generation of vasoactive substances is possible during such therapy. Another possible reaction is the leakage of pyrogens or sensitizing substances from the modules. Clinical manifestation such as temperature elevations, chills, hypo- and hypertension have been observed and reported [21, 23]. Of the plasma fractionation schemes employed or being designed, we believe that the techniques of nonbiologic (contains no immunologically active entity that if it is leached or interacts with the blood may promote an immunologic response) is to be preferred where clinical applicable.

While the biomodulating influence has centered on the humoral modulating effects of plasmapheresis, it should be emphasized that cellular modulation may also occur. Numerous reports have pointed out the effects of humoral factors and their changes on cellular counts and functions. It has been shown that phagocytic function can be increased and that effects on lymphocytes as measured by mitogen studies and ratios of cell populations pre- to post-plasmapheresis may be produced [22]. Thus, the biological influences of plasmapheresis therapies affect not only such humoral components as proteins, antibodies, acute phase reactants, serum blocking factors, and complement, but also the cellular components such as white blood cells, most notably the lymphocytes, phagocytes, and platelets. While various studies on select disease states have shown the influence of humoral factors on cellular changes and functional improvements with solute removal, the effects of cellular improvement are not necessarily due solely to solute removal, but may relate to the procedure itself [11].

Future direction

One important area of progress in apheresis is the further development of technology. Technology for more selective and optimal removal of pathologically relevant molecules and cells from body will become more refined in clinical use of plasmapheresis through on-line plasma treatment and the development of selective and specific adsorbents. Simple plasma separation will be replaced with more selective removal technologies.

Plasma fractionation by membrane fractionation or adsorbents are not yet widely accepted in the disease states treated by plasmapheresis, although a few disease states are being treated by these technologies in increasing numbers. Perhaps better membranes or innovative filtration techniques will permit IgG and albumin fractionation and thereby enable a more widespread application of plasma fractionation [24].

The development of on-line plasmapheresis by membrane fractionation and adsorption techniques emphasizes the importance for a greater understanding of the pathogenetic role of circulating agents in the blood. Further research into the kinetics of pathogenetic substances and blood-material interaction (biomodulation effect) and the more conscious selection of patient and disease stage is also required before plasmapheresis techniques for their selective removal can be designed for maximum efficacy and clinical effects.

As apheresis related technology, the concept of adoptive immunotherapy, adopting the organism's own body to fight the disease, and leukocytapheresis have been aggressively pursued in recent years with regards to cell therapy [25]. The adaptive immunotherapy approach and leukocytapheresis require further optimization of the techniques for bulk cell processing and the separation of specific cell types to make it more practical and effective. Perhaps combined with other agents such as immunosuppressive drug therapy or if further refinement of cell separation can be lead to selective removals of only pathogenic lymphocytes, lymphocytapheresis and these adoptive immunotherapy might eventually become a practical and useful treatment modality.

In the future, there must be clear evidence of the efficacy of plasmapheresis, sufficient information to delineate its role properly in the total treatment armamentarium for the disorder, and definition of the successful treatment schedule [5].

The wave of the future is cost containment in medicine. Cost effectiveness will be possible for plasmapheresis to become an acceptable and established therapy for a wide range of diseases. The objective of plasmapheresis is to reduce or stop the progression of end-stage disease. Through biochemical and immunological modulation by apheresis treatment technologies, it is hoped that the number of end-stage patients will be reduced.

References

[1] PATTEN, E.: Therapeutic plasmapheresis and plasma exchange. *CRC* 23: 147-175 (1986).
[2] MALCHESKY, P. S., T. HORIUCHI, J. J. LEWANDOWSKI, Y. NOSÉ: Membrane plasma separation and the on-line plasma treatment by membrane. *J. Membrane Sci.* 44: 55-88 (1989).
[3] VANGELISTA, A., G. M. FRASCA, V. BONOMINI: Parameters for indication of plasmapheresis and the interpretation of the results. *Clinical Nephrology* 26 (Suppl. 1): 64-69 (1986).
[4] SUTTON, D. M. C., R. C. NAIR, G. ROCK: Complications of plasma exchange. *Transfusion* 29: 124-127 (1989).
[5] COUNCIL REPORT: Current Status of Therapeutic Plasmapheresis and related Techniques. Report of the AMA Panel on Therapeutic Plasmapheresis. *JAMA* 253(6): 819-825 (1985).
[6] ROTHWEL, R. S., P. DAVIS, P. GORDON: A controlled study of plasma exchange in the treatment of severe rheumatoid arthritis. *Arthritis Rheum* 23: 785-790 (1980).
[7] WALLACE, D., D. GOLDFINGER, D. LOWE: A double-blind controlled study of lymphoplasmapheresis vs sham apheresis in rheumatoid arthritis. *N. Engl. J. Med.* 306: 1406-1410 (1982).
[8] DWOSH, I. L., A. R. GILES, P. M. FORD: Plasmapheresis therapy in rheumatoid arthritis: a controlled double-blind, crossover trial. *N. Engl. J. Med.* 308(19): 1124-1128 (1983).
[9] Clinical applications of therapeutic apheresis report of the clinical applications committee American Society for apheresis. *J. Clin. Apheresis* 3: 192-252 (1986).
[10] NOSÉ, Y., H. E. KAMBIC, F. MATSUBARA: Introduction to Therapeutic Apheresis, pp. 1-22. In: NOSÉ, Y., et al. (eds.): Plasmapheresis, 1983.
[11] MALCHESKY, P. S., Y. NOSÉ: Biomodulation Effects of Extracorporeal Circulation in Apheresis. *Sem. Hemat.* 26(2), Suppl. 1: 42-51 (1989).
[12] REILLY, R. W.: Issues and trends affecting plasma selection for use in further manufacture: worldwide. *J. Clin. Apheresis* 4: 85-88 (1988).
[13] MALCHESKY, P. S., J. D. CLOUGH: Cryoglobulinemia: properties, prevalence in disease and removal. *Cleve Clin. Q.* 52: 175-189 (1985).
[14] MALCHESKY, P. S., J. W. SMITH, A. KOO, J. D. CLOUGH, Y. NOSÉ: Uncontrolled trial of cryofiltration in rheumatoid arthritis. *J. Clin. Apheresis* 4: 158-165 (1988).
[15] MALCHESKY, P. S., Y. NOSÉ: Cryoprocesses for macromolecule separation, pp. 200-212. In: LYSAGHT, M. J., et al. (eds.): Plasma separation and plasma fractionation, 1983.
[16] SAKAMOTO, S., P. S. MALCHESKY, J. W. SMITH, Y. NOSÉ: Apheresis: clinical response in patients unresponsive to conventional therapy. *Trans. Am. Soc. Artif. Int. Org.* 31: 704-789 (1985).
[17] MALCHESKY, P. S., Y. ASANUMA, Y. NOSÉ: On-line separation of macromolecules by membrane filtration with cryogelation. *Art. Organs.* 4: 205-207 (1980).
[18] CLOUGH, J. D., E. P. PAGANINI: Therapeutic Plasmapheresis Current status and future prospects. *Postgrad. Med.* 75(7): 77-84 (1984).
[19] AGISHI, T.: Therapeutic membrane Plasmapheresis, pp. 17-24. In: ODA, T., et al. (eds.): Proceedings of the first International Congress of the World Apheresis Association: Therapeutic plasmapheresis (VI). ISAO Press: Cleveland 1986.
[20] KOTTEKE, B. A., A. PINEDA, M. T. CASE, A. M. ORSUZAR, K. A. BRZYS: Hypercholesterolemia and atherosclerosis; present and future therapy including LDL-apheresis. *J. Clin. Apheresis* 4: 35-46 (1988).
[21] BEHM, E., P. IVANOVICH, H. KLINKMAN: Selective and specific adsorbents for medical therapy. *Int. J. Artif. Organs* 12(1): 1-10 (1989).
[22] YAMAZAKI, Z.: Extracorporeal Immunoabsorption. In: ODA, T.: Plasmapheresis (VI), 1986.
[23] SHUMAK, K. H., G. A. ROCK: Therapeutic Plasma Exchange. *N. Engl. J. Med.* 65: 564-565 (1984).
[24] SAMTLEBEN, W., M. J. LYSAGHT, H. J. GURLAND: Therapeutic Plasma Exchange: Achievements versus Expectations. *Contr. Nephrology* 44: 223-235 (1985).
[25] ROSENBERG, S. A., W. D. TERRY: Passive immunotherapy of cancer in animals and man. *Adv. Cancer Res.* 25: 3232-3388 (1977).
[26] WOOD, L., P. JACOBS: The effect of serial therapeutic plasmapheresis on platelet count, coagulation factors, plasma immunoglobulin and complement. *J. Clin. Apheresis* 3: 124-128 (1986).

Extracorporeal LDL-Adsorption Treatment in Hyperlipidemia: Clinical Applications and New Developments

TH. BOSCH

Abstract

Clinical LDL-adsorption has made overwhelming progress in recent years. Thus, immunoadsorption with polyclonal anti-LDL-antibodies and chemoadsorption using the dextransulfate system have been applied successfully for selective LDL-removal in routine clinical plasma treatment of hypercholesterolemic patients suffering from coronary artery disease. Clinical pilot studies showed good results using immunoadsorption with anti-LDL-F(ab)-columns. Promising laboraty results have been achieved using immunoadsorption with monoclonal LDL-antibodies, polyacrylate/fractogel and macroporous cellulose. While these systems need a primary separation step for cells and plasma, the integrated plasma separation/adsorption device and the LDL-hemoperfusion modul using E 280590 can even treat whole blood. Thus, these systems hold a great promise for the future.

Introduction

Since the introduction of plasma therapy into the treatment of hyperlipidemia by Thompson in 1967 [1], rapid progress has been made in the field of extracorporeal plasma treatment for this indication. Several treatment modalities have been applied: simple plasma exchange [1], double filtration at room temperature [2] and thermofiltration at 37-42° C [3], LDL-precipitation by heparin at pH 5.12 [4] or by dextransulfate in the presence of Ca^{2+} [5]. The present article focuses on the methods of LDL-adsorption which were developed in recent years.

LDL-adsorption using anti-LDL-ligands

Polyclonal anti-LDL-antibodies

First published by Stoffel and Demant in 1981, this system was later introduced into the clinical routine treatment of patients suffering from severe hypercholesterolemia [6, 7]. In principle, heterologous polyclonal antibodies against human LDL are immobilized on sepharose 4B. Plasma is run over one of two parallel immunoadsorbers containing about 400 ml of gel. Once the column has been saturated with LDL, the apheresis machine (Baxter, Munich, FRG) automatically switches to the second fresh adsorber while the first is regenerated on-line by glycine/HCI, PBS buffer and saline. Columns are reused for about 50 times in the same patient. Thus, strict microbiological tests for bacterial and pyrogen contaminations have to be performed prior to each treatment. The columns are stored at 4° C using NaN_3 as additive. LDL elimination is highly selective with 58-70 % LDL-C, 25-30 % HDL-C, 51 % triglyceride, 22 % Lp(a) and 25-32 % fibrinogen reduction (reduction = $(1 - C_{pre}/C_{post}) \times 100\%$) after treatment of about one patient plasma volume [8, 9]. More than 3000 treatments have been performed using this system and the first study of regression of atherosclerosis by means of extracorporeal LDL-apheresis in ten patients was published by Hombach et al. in 1986 [10].

LDL-immunoadsorption using anti-LDL-F(ab) columns

In 1986, Riesen et al. [11] published their results using an 800 ml LDL-immunoadsorber containing heterologous anti-LDL-F(ab)-fragments immobilized on sepharose CL 4B. At the bottom of the column, a “filter” of 50 mg of human LDL immobilized on sepharose is attached in order to adsorb any anti-LDL-F(ab) antibodies desorbed from the column thus preventing them to enter into the systemic circulation of the patient. LDL-adsorption capacity of the column amounts to 20 g cholesterol. According to the authors, anti-LDL-F(ab) columns offer the advantage of lower immunogenicity of F(ab)-fragments in comparison to complete anti-LDL-antibodies. Treating about one patient plasma volume results in 77 % LDL-C, 28 % HDL-C, 50 % triglyceride, 81 % apo B and 40 % Apo A II reduction. This system was applied successfully in a clinical trial with a small number of patients.

LDL-immunoadsorption using monoclonal anti-LDL-antibodies

In 1986, Koren et al. [12] described the formation of monoclonal anti-LDL-antibodies by a mouse-hybridoma cell-line. These were immobilized and used for LDL-immunoadsorption in vitro with good results. Pokrovsky [13] reported on a clinical pilot study using monoclonal immunoadsorbers in FH-patients with good results. One of the alleged advantages of these columns is the easy regeneration of the columns due to the homogeneous nature of the antibodies which could result in longer life-time of the adsorbers due to milder regeneration conditions. Further trials are warranted in order to allow the assessment of the clinical potential of the columns in the future.

LDL-chemoadsorption using dextransulfate

In 1985, Yokoyama et al. [14] reported on clinical results of LDL-adsorption in FH-patients using dextransulfate immobilized on cellulose beads. Meanwhile this system has been developed to clinical maturity and is being applied in many centers all over the world. In principle, plasma is treated much in the same way as described above for the anti-LDL-antibody system using two parallel adsorbers (containing 150 ml gel each) which can be regenerated on-line by hyperosmolar saline. All the components of the extracorporeal material are single-use products. Reduction percentages are 60-64 % for LDL-C, 15-17 % for HDL-C, 50 % for triglycerides, 15 % for Lp(a) and 10-50 % for fibrinogen [8, 15]. Nonspecific loss of proteins is negligible.

Moreover, complement components generated in the process of plasma separation using hollow fibre moduls are also adsorbed with high efficiency.

In contrast to anti-LDL-antibody columns which work on the principle of an antigen (apo B coating LDL)- antibody (anti-LDL-antibody immobilized on sepharose) reaction, chemoadsorption by dextransulfate is based on an electrostatic ionic interaction between the polyanion dextransulfate and the polycation apo B.

LDL-adsorption using polyacrylate

In 1988, Thies et al. [16] described LDL-adsorption from plasma onto polyacrylate immobilized on fractogel. Successful in vitro experiments were followed by perfusion of 2.5 l plasma through a 200 ml adsorber in three sheep.

LDL-C and triglycerides were decreased significantly, while HDL-C, AT III, fibrinogen and calcium levels remained constant. No application of this system in patients has been described so far.

LDL-adsorption using macroporous cellulose

Behm et al. reported on the astonishingly selective binding properties of a specially prepared macroporous cellulose for LDL-adsorption [17]. This cheap material was tested in vitro with good results and the authors hypothesized that this effect was due to a molecular sieving of the larger LDL particles within the macroporous internal structure of the cellulose while HDL particles could diffuse freely in and out of the cellulose. Moreover, hydrogen bonding and/or hydrophobic interactions as possible binding mechanisms of LDL-adsorption were discussed.

Integrated plasma separation and adsorption devices

This new system is based on the observation that a plasma bypass flow is established in the plasma compartment of a hollow fibre separator modul even if the plasma compartment entry and exit are closed. This is due to plasma filtration across the hollow fibre membrane in the first half of its length and backfiltration from the plasma compartment into the hollow fibre in the second half. Smolik et al. [18] filled the plasma compartment with dextransulfate/cellulose beads and could attain a good selective LDL-adsorption from whole blood. This is a very interesting approach because the treatment of whole blood does away with the primary separation step of cells and plasma and could thus simplify the process of LDL-adsorption substantially. Experiments were performed in an ex-vivo single-pass set-up in our laboratory. Cholesterol adsorption capacity ranged from 5-10 mg/g gel, and HDL-C was recovered almost completely. However, these promising results await further clinical corroboration in patient trials.

LDL-hemoperfusion using E 280590

This new material (Fresenius, Bad Homburg, FRG) consists of a surface-modified polyacrylate matrix and was recently tested for biocompatibility in our laboraty. Whole blood of healthy donors was passed through the adsorption column in an ex-vivo single-pass mode. According to the manufacturer, LDL-binding capacity was 8-10 mg LDL-C/g, while HDL-C was not adsorbed. Our data [19] show surprisingly low thrombogenicity of this material which make this system a promising candidate for LDL-adsorption from whole blood in a hemoperfusion setting. Again, clinical application in the future will show whether this material will prove to be of clinical benefit in patients.

References

[1] THOMPSON, G. R., R. LOWENTHAL, N. B. MYANT: Plasma exchange in the management of homozygous familial hypercholesterolemia. *Lancet* 1: 1208-1211 (1975).

[2] KOCHINKE, F., H. VON BAEYER, I. SCHWANER, R. SCHWERDTFEGER: Comparison of plasma fractionation filters and filtration techniques in the clinical practice of LDL-apheresis. *Trans. Am. Soc. Artif. Organs* 32: 388-391 (1986).

[3] NOSÉ, Y., M. USAMI, P. S. MALCHESKY, M. EMURA, T. HORIUCHI, H. SAKAMOTO, J. W. SMITH: Clinical thermofiltration: initial application. *Artif. Organs* 9: 425-427 (1985).

[4] EISENHAUER, T., V. W. ARMSTRONG, H. WIELAND, C. FUCHS, F. SCHELER, D. SEIDEL: Selective removal of LDL by precipitation at low pH: first clinical application of the HELP system. *Klin. Wochenschr.* 65: 161-168 (1987).

[5] ANTWILER, G. D., P. C. DAU, D. D. LOBDELL: Reduction of low-density lipoprotein with dextran sulfate in patients with familial hypercholesterolemia. *J. Clin. Apheresis* 4: 18-29 (1988).

[6] STOFFEL, W., T. DEMANT: Selective removal of apolipoprotein B-containing serum lipoproteins from blood plasma. *Proc. Natl. Acad. Sci. USA* 78: 611-615 (1981).

[7] BORBERG, H., A. GACZKOWSKI, V. HOMBACH, K. OETTE, W. STOFFEL: Treatment of familial hypercholesterolemia by means of specific immunoadsorption. *J. Clin. Apheresis* 4: 59-65 (1988).

[8] KELLER, CH.: Extrakorporale Lipoproteinelimination – Indikation und Differentialtherapie. *Dialyse-Journal* 32: 15-20 (1990).

[9] BORBERG, H., C. BODE, L. MATTELE, K. OETTE, M. TAUCHERT, W. STOFFEL: LDL-Apheresis in hypercholesterolemic patients: Technical and clinical aspects, pp. 266-271. In: GURLAND, H. J., M. J. LYSAGHT (eds.): Plasma separation and fractionation. Karger: Basel 1983.

[10] HOMBACH, V., H. BORBERG, A. GACZKOWSKI, K. OETTE, W. STOFFEL: Regression der Koronarsklerose bei familiärer Hypercholesterinämie IIa durch spezifische LDL-Apherese. *Dt. Med. Wschr.* 111: 1709-1715 (1986).

[11] RIESEN, W. F., C. IMHOF, E. STURZENEGGER, C. DESCOEUDRES, R. MORDASINI, O. H. OETLIKER: Behandlung einer Hypercholesterinämie durch extrakorporale Immunadsorption. *Schweiz. Med. Wschr.* 116: 8-11 (1986).

[12] KOREN, E., C. KNIGHT-GIBSON, G. WEN, L. DE BAULT, P. ALAUPOVIC: Characterization of a monoclonal antibody that binds equally to all apolipoprotein and lipoprotein forms of human plasma apolipoprotein B. II. Isolation of apolipoprotein B – containing lipoproteins from human plasma. *Biochim. Biophys. Acta* 876: 101-107 (1986).

[13] POKROVSKY, S.: LDL-apheresis using monoclonal anti-LDL-antibodies. Presentation at the XVI. ESAO Congress, Brussels, Sept. 14, 1989.

[14] YOKOYAMA, S., R. HAYASHI, M. SATANI, A. YAMAMOTO: Selective removal of LDL by plasmapheresis in familial hypercholesterolemia. *Arteriosclerosis* 5: 613-622 (1985).

[15] BOSCH, TH., M. BLUMENSTEIN, U. DENDORFER, W. SAMTLEBEN, B. SCHMIDT, H. J. GURLAND: Klinische LDL-Adsorption an Dextransulfat mit automatischer on-line Adsorberregeneration bei Hyperlipoproteinämie, pp. 38-51. In: GURLAND, H. J., K. M. KOCH, W. SCHOEPPE, P. SCIGALLA (eds.): Innovative Aspekte der Klinischen Medizin, Band 1. Springer: Heidelberg 1989.

[16] THIES, K., S. A. PRIGENT, C. C. HEUCK: Selective removal of LDL from plasma by polyacrylate-coated fractogel in vitro and in experimental extracorporeal perfusion. *Artif. Organs* 12: 320-324 (1988).

[17] BEHM, E., F. LOTH, D. TOEWE, O. ZSCHÖRNIG, B. ERNST, H. KLINKMANN: Low density lipoprotein binding by macroporous bead cellulose. *Biomed. Biochim. Acta* 48: 829-837 (1989).

[18] SMOLIK, G., B. SCHMIDT, U. BAURMEISTER, M. HAMPE, H. J. GURLAND: New design of an integral device for absorption from whole blood (Abstract). *Artif. Organs* 13: 368 (1989).

[19] SCHMIDT, B.: Ex-vivo evaluation of biocompatibility. Presentation at the Xth Int. Symp. on Hemoperfusion, Adsorbents and Immobilized Reactants, Rome, Sept. 24, 1990.

The Treatment of Multiple Sclerosis: First Results of a Three-Armed Study Comparing Immunoadsorption, Plasma Exchange and Steroids

E. SCHMITT, E. BEHM, F. BUDDENHAGEN, B. HITZSCHKE, M. KRACHT, G. KUNDT, H. MEYER-RIENECKER, B. OSTEN, M. PALM, R. WINKLER, H. KLINKMANN

Abstract

Up to now 17 patients entered the study suffering from acute relapsing or chronically progressive multiple sclerosis. The duration of multiple sclerosis averaged approximately 10 years. Patients were randomized for allocation into three groups. All patients received steroids. Immunoadsorption was performed in group 1. Plasma exchange treatments were performed in group 2. Mono-therapy with prednisolone 60 mg/day was administered to group 3.

The quantitative scoring scales of multiple sclerosis showed a poor effect in the steroid group. Marked improvement was obtained for at least three months in the immunoadsorption and similarly in the plasma exchange groups. A more pronounced effect was achieved in the functional systems: Prednisolone provided a short and questionable effect. There was a clear improvement in the plasma exchange group and even more in the immunoadsorption group after two weeks which was maintained over several months. Best results were obtained in the relapsing patients. There were no side effects in the immunoadsorption group. In plasma exchange two patients developed "weakness" and one a gastric ulcer due to steroids.

The authors speculate that a reduction of complement activity by 75 % in both, the immunoadsorption and the plasma exchange groups is responsible for the beneficial effect.

Introduction

There is reason to believe that immune processes play an important role in the pathogenesis of multiple sclerosis (MS). In the acute form there is said to be an altered blood brain barrier. Therefore, the removal of pathogenetically relevant substances, whatever they might be out of the circulation provides a therapeutic chance in MS predominantly in acute patients. When we started our trial in 1985, P. C. Dau [1], P. Höcker [2] and B. O. Khatri [3] had published encouraging results in the PE treatment of MS. At that time, there were also some reports on the successful application of the immunoadsorbent column IM-P made by Shibuya [4].

Patients and Methods

Only patients with clinically definite MS which were chronically progressive or in an acute exacerbation were included in the study. They were allocated into the treatment groups by use of a computerized blocked randomization program, based on three parameters:

1. Sex,
2. Age at onset of the disease – below 30 years or older – and
3. Mode of activity – chronic progression or acute relapse. Before entering the study patients gave their informed consent. The study comprises three groups:

1. **Group P:** Patients were treated with prednisolone only: 60 mg i.v. per day over a period of one week. Then the dose was reduced to 30 mg orally which was administered for another four weeks.
2. **Group PE:** The steroid therapy was the same. Four plasma exchange treatments were performed within one week. The exchange volume was 50 ml/kg body weight at each session using 5 % albumin in Ringer's as replacement solution.
3. **Group IA:** Steroids were administered following the same protocol. Within one week we performed plasma sorption four times making use of the Plasmaflo and the immunoadsorbent column Immunsorba PH-350, both from Asahi Medical, Tokyo, Japan. The plasma volume processed through the column was also 50 ml/kg body weight at each session.

It should be noted that the ethics committee did not accept our proposal to have a group with sham apheresis.

Two experienced neurologists carried out clinical examinations before starting the study, after two weeks, three months later and after one year. The degree of impairment in the functional systems (FS) was measured according to Kurtzke. The measurement of the neurological impairments was done by means of the expanded disability status scale (EDSS) also after Kurtzke. Neurologists and patients were blinded as to what kind of extracorporeal treatment was done. The dialysis physicians did not receive any actual information about the neurological examinations. Up to now 19 patients have entered the study. There were eight males and 11 females, 11 had acute exacerbation and eight patients suffered from the chronic progressive form. Here we present preliminary results with an amount of cases being too small for statistical evaluation.

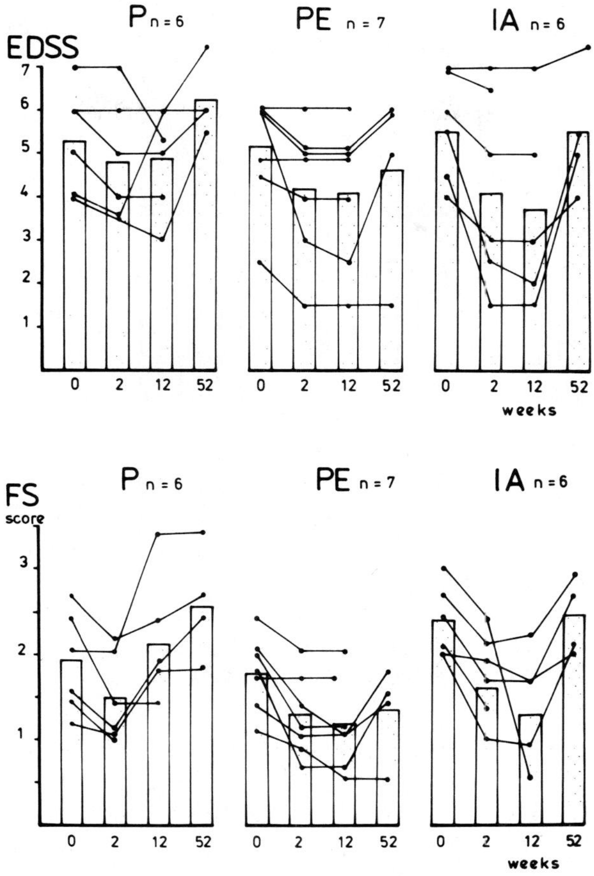

Fig. 1. Neurological findings in the EDSS and the FS after Kurtzke in the groups P, PE and IA.

Results

When looking firstly at the EDSS results one can see that after two weeks there is a poor effect by the prednisolone therapy. A marked improvement, however, was obtained for at least three months in the PE and in the IA group. The columns indicate mean values of all patients and the lines show the results of single cases. A more pronounced effect was achieved in the functional systems. It is demonstrated that prednisolone alone provides a short and questionable effect. In the PE group and even more clearly in the IA group there is a significant improvement after two weeks which was maintained over several months. Generally, the best results were obtained in the acute relapse patients. After one year we found deterioration in all groups (Fig. 1). No side-effects were observed in the IA and the prednisolone

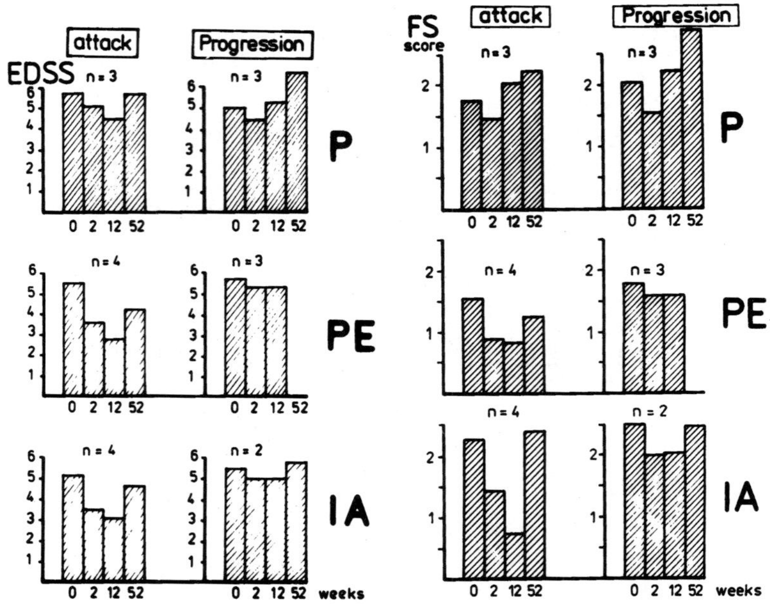

Fig. 2. Different results in the EDSS and the FS by discriminating between acute relapsers and chronic progressive patients in the groups P, PE and IA.

group. Two of the PE patients developed weakness for a few days and one had to be operated for a gastric ulcer due to the steroids. We also made an attempt to analyse our data in order to find out where we got the best or poorest results. When considering the columns in Figure 2 there was no effect at 12 weeks in the drug treated patients. PE provides no benefit in the chronic progressive patients whereas there was a certain beneficial effect in the acute ones.

The best results were obtained in the acute relapse patients treated with immunoadsorption. In trying to explain similar effects of the different extracorporeal treatments we analyzed the immunoglobulins and complement behavior. In Figure 3 we can show in the upper part that PE reduces the immunoglobulins A, G and M and fibrinogen by about 75 % of the pretreatment values. In the case of IA there is only a slight decrease of these proteins by about 15-20 %. When we turned to consideration of the hemolytic activity of both the classical and alternate pathway, we found them to be significantly reduced by the PE and also by IA. In Figure 4 the CH 50 levels of the classical pathway before and after each treatment are connected by a line. One can see a reduction of the complement activity by both, IA and PE, by approximately 75 % at each session. We would like to speculate that behind this reduction of the complement activity we can find the reason for the beneficial effect of the both treatments.

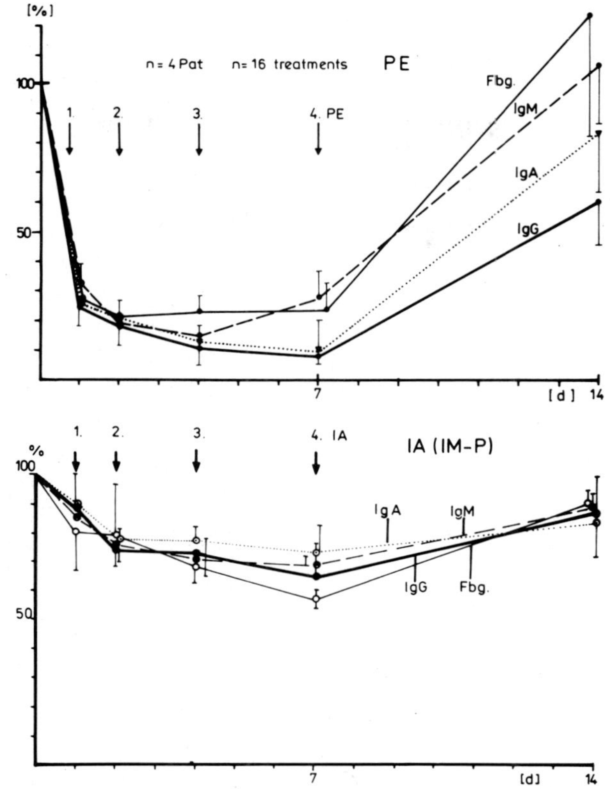

Fig. 3. Changes (post treatment) in fibrinogen and immunoglobulins A, G and M in PE and IA.

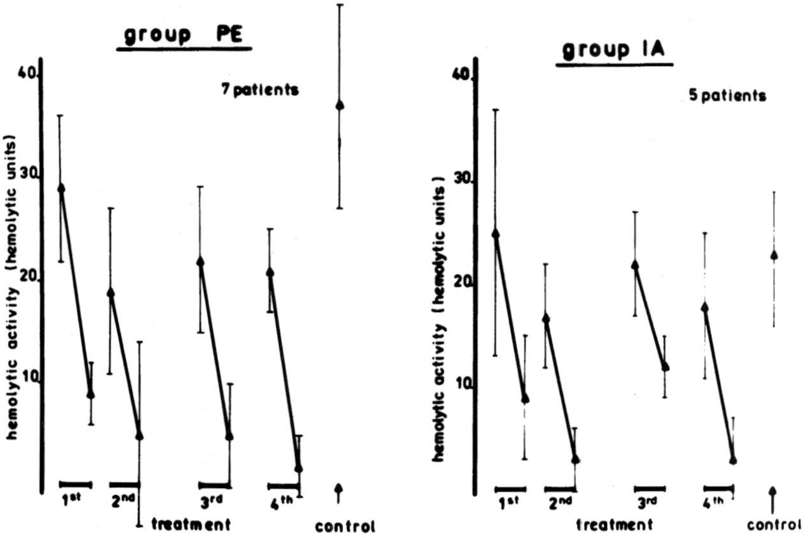

Fig. 4. CH 50 before and after each treatment of PE (left) and IA (right).

Conclusion

We would like to state that

- In our opinion the PE and IA treatments are more effective than steroids alone, especially in cases with acute exacerbation.
- When comparing IA and PE we would prefer IA because of the lack of side effects and a similar or even better therapeutic effect.
- The therapeutic effect seems to be achieved by the reduction of complement activity.
- The activity of MS can be influenced for only a limited period of time.
- To expect a long-term effect after a one-week treatment is not realistic.
- The patients of our study are treated again when a relapse occurs.
- With respect to our results it appears justified to apply a chronic IA therapy in order to prevent deterioration. A controlled study should be initiated in order to find some evidence for this speculation.

References

[1] DAU, P. C., R. G. MILLER, E. H. DENYS: Experience with plasmapheresis in 153 neurologic patients. *Int. J. Art. Organs* 5: 37-46 (1982).

[2] HÖCKER, P., V. STELLAMOR, K. SUMMER, M. MANN: Plasmaexchange and lymphocytapheresis in multiple sclerosis. *Int. J. Artif. Organs* 7: 39-42 (1984).

[3] KHATRI, B. O., M. P. MCQUILLEN, G. J. HARRINGTON, D. SCHMOLL, R. G. HOFFMANN: Chronic progressive multiple sclerosis: Double-blind controlled study of plasmapheresis in patients taking immunosuppressive drugs. *Neurology* 35: 312-319.

[4] SHIBUYA, N., K. NAGASATO, K. SHIBAYAMA, H. KANAZAWA: Immunoabsorption therapy in neurologic disorders: myasthenia gravis, multiple sclerosis and Guillain-Barré-Syndrome, pp. 122-128. In: ODA, T., Y. SHIOKAWA, N. INOUE (eds.): Proceedings of the 1st International Congress of the World Apheresis Association. ISAO Press: Cleveland 1987.

Can a Patient Get Accustomed to a Special Type of Dialyzer Membrane?

R. SCHMIDT, R. BAMBAUER, B. OSTEN, P. IVANOVICH, H. KLINKMANN

Introduction

Anaphylactoid reactions when using a new type of dialyzer have been reported many times [1-3]. Symptoms ranging from mild flushing, sweating, urticaria, headache, backache through moderate distress with vomiting, diarrhea, shivers, chest pain and tachycardia to life-threatening complications as severe bronchospasm, hypotension and cardiac arrest can be observed and have been termed Hypersensitivity Syndrome or First Use Syndrome. Patients show these symptoms within a few minutes of the blood initially returning from the hemodialyzer to the patients circulation, typically within as little as 1-5 minutes. The pathogenesis of this syndrom is unknown. Allergy to ethylene oxide (ETO), a chemical used in sterilizing many of the involved dialyzers, has been implicated [4]. Components present in dialyzers from the processing may be associated with toxic effects [5-7]. After the contact of the blood with the dialyzer membrane the patient's blood reacts causing activation of plasma complement during hemodialysis depending on the type of membrane [8, 9]. Cuprophan dialyzers are known to be associated with a higher degree of complement activation [10, 11]. Conversely, membranes consisting of cellulose acetate, acrylonitrile, polysulfone and polypropylene show a much lesser degree of complement activation [11-13]. The incidence of the First Use Syndrome was frequently related to a high degree of complement activation.

In a previous study [14] 13 patients out of the regular dialysis program who were routinely dialyzed with cellulose acetate hemodialyzers participated in a blinded cross over study comparing dialyzers with Cuprophan or cellulose acetate membranes. Dialyzers of comparable surface area and configuration were used. The 13 patients accustomed to cellulose acetate dialyzers were switched to a Cuprophan dialyzer. Five out of the 13 patients developed severe clinical symptoms in the sense of hypersensitivity syndrome. Complement activation (especially C3a) was found three times higher in Cuprophan hemodialysis than in cellulose acetate hemodialysis. The drop in neutrophils showed the same behavior as complement activation. From these results we concluded that time:

- Cellulose acetate membranes are better tolerated than Cuprophan membranes.
- The degree of complement activation and the drop of neutrophils are important determinants for dialysis membranes.

But looking at the individual results we recognized that the patients with the most severe clinical complications did not show the highest degree of complement activation. There was no correlation between complement activation and drop of neutrophils and the severeness of clinical symptoms.

Methods

A new dialyzer (MLW 1.8 m^2/GDR) containing a dialysis membrane of regenerated cellulose was introduced and had to be tested for efficacy and hemocompatibility. 42 RDT patients accustomed to the CD-Medical dialyzer (CDAK 1.8 m^2), that contains also a dialysis membrane of regenerated cellulose, were treated with the new dialyzer and 127 hemodialysis courses were observed carefully. Clearances, ultrafiltration rate, drop of neutrophils after 15 minutes of treatment and clinical symptoms were investigated and recorded. Both dialyzers had been sterilized with ethylene oxide. Priming and rinsing procedure had been performed in an identical way.

Table 1. Clinical Symptons in the Initial Phase of Hemodialysis (MLW 1.8).

Back pain	1
Headache	2
Chest pain	1
Heat	4
Shivers	1
Irritated Taste	1
Coldness	3
Strangle feeling	1
Total (n = 127)	14 = 11 %

Results

14 patients experienced clinical symptoms, listed in Table 1, 5-15 minutes after starting hemodialysis with the new dialyzer MLW 1.8 m^2. 11 patients showed their clinical complications in the first treatment with the new dialyzer and three patients during the second hemodialysis with the MLW 1.8 m^2 dialyzer. Table 2 shows the drop of neutrophils after 15 minutes hemodialysis with the dialyzer CDAK 1.8 m^2 and the MLW 1.8 m^2 as well. During CDAK-hemodialysis the neutrophils dropped to 66.6 % ± 4.8 % from the initial level after 15 minutes treatment and during MLW-hemodialysis neutrophils decreased to 72.2 % ±5.1 % after 15 minutes of hemodialysis. The 14 patients with clinical symptoms showed an average drop of neutrophils to 69.3 % ± 6.8 % from the initial level.

Discussion

In our study both CDAK 1.8 m^2 and MLW 1.8 m^2 dialyzers were associated with a comparable degree of leukopenia after 15 minutes hemodialysis treatment. On the other hand we observed with the MLW 1.8 m^2 hemodialysis clinical complications in 14 patients and did not with the CDAK 1.8 m^2 treatment. The 14 patients with clinical symptoms did not show a higher degree of leukopenia. It has to be mentioned that these 14 patients did tolerate the new MLW 1.8 m^2 dialyzer without any problems having been exposed to it for four weeks. Both CDAK 1.8 m^2 and MLW 1.8 m^2 dialyzers contain a hemodialysis membrane of regenerated cellulose but the chemical way of processing is different. The CDAK-membrane is produced via cellulose acetate and the MLW-membrane via cellulose xanthongenate. Since both membranes show a similar degree in drop of neutrophils we can assume a comparable hemocompatibility. The only explanation for the clinical complications when using a new dialyzer with similar hemocompatibility of its membrane is a toxic effect. It is well known in medicine that a patient can get accustomed to increasing doses of a toxin without getting troubles. Complement activation and drop of neutrophils occur during every hemodialysis without creating problems. A very high percentage of hemodialysis centers are dialyzing with Cuprophan dialyzers without any complications.

Our observations suggest that at least a part of the reasons of the hypersensitivity syndrome has to be referred to toxicity. Patients seem to be able to get accustomed to a type of dialyzer with its special membrane and chemicals remaining from processing. The dominating role of complement activation in causing a hypersensitivity syndrome seems to be doubtful.

Table 2. Decrease of Neutrophils after 15 minutes. Hemodialysis (n = 15).

CDAK 1.8	MLW 1.8
(regenerated Cellulose via Cellulose Acetate)	(regenerated Cellulose via Cellulose Xantogenate)
66.6 %	73.2 %
±4.8 %	±5.1 %

References

[1] NICHOLLS, A.: Hypersensitivity to Hemodialysis: The United Kingdom Experience. *Artif. Organs* 11: 87-89 (1987).

[2] SCHMIDT, R., B. OSTEN: Klinische Aspekte beim Einsatz der Künstlichen Niere. *Z. gesamte inn. Med.* 309-313 (1986).

[3] VILLARROEL, F., A. CIARKOWSKI: A Survey on hypersensitivity reactions in hemodialysis. *Artif. Organs* 9: 231-238 (1985).

[4] BOMMER, J., E. RITZ: Ethylene oxide as a major cause of anaphylactoid reactions in dialysis. *Artif. Organs* 11: 111-117 (1987).

[5] DAUGIRDAS, J. T., L. D. POTEMPA, V. C. GANDHI, D. NGOCLAN, P. IVANOVICH, T. S. ING: Plate, Coil, and Hollow-Fiber Cuprammonium Cellulose Dialyzers: Discrepancy Between Incidence of Anaphylactic Reactions and Degree of Complement Activation. *Artif. Organs* 11(2): 140-143 (1987).

[6] KJELLSTRAND, C., A. ALFREY, J. EATON, E. FRIEDMANN, H. GINN, A. HULL, D. OGDEN: Toxicity of materials and medications used in dialysis. *Trans. Am. Soc. Artif. Int. Org.* 24: 764-769 (1978).

[7] MAURICE, F., J. RIVORY, J. BOUSQUET, F. MICHEL: Anaphylactic shock with formaldehyde (Abstract). *J. Allergyclin. Immunol* 74: 209 (1985).

[8] BAURMEISTER, U., W. VIENKEN, W. ANSORGE, A. LUTTRELL: Cellulosic versus Synthetic Membranes: A Reasonable Comparison? *Artif. Organs* 13(1): 52-57 (1989).

[9] KLINKMANN, H.: Biocompatibility Problems in Membrane Separation Processes, pp. 17-23. In: BAMBAUER, R., P. S. MALCHESKY, D. FALKENHAGEN (eds.): Therapeutic Plasma Exchange and Selective Plasma Separation. Schattauer: Stuttgart-New York 1987.

[10] CHENOWETH, D. E., A. CHEUNG, L. W. HENDERSON: Anaphylatoxin formation during hemodialysis: effects of different dialyzer membranes. *Kidney Int.* 24: 764 (1983).

[11] HAKIM, R., E. LOWRIE: Effect of dialyzer reuse on leukopenia, hypoxemia and total hemolyctic complement system. *Trans. Am. Soc. Artif. Int. Org.* 26: 159-164 (1980).

[12] CHENOWETH, D. E.: Complement activation during hemodialysis: clinical observations, proposed mechanisms, and theoretical implications. *Art. Organs* 8: 281-287 (1984).

[13] KLINKMANN, H., D. FALKENHAGEN, J. H. COURTNEY: Clinical relevance of biocompatibility. "The material cannot be divorced from the device". *Nefrologia* 7, Suppl. 3: 13-20 (1987).

[14] IVANOVICH, P., D. E. CHENOWETH, R. SCHMIDT, H. KLINKMANN, L. A. BOXER, H. S. JACOB, D. HAMMERSCHMIDT: Symptoms and activation of granulocytes and complement with two dialysis membranes. *Kidney Int.* 24: 758-763 (1983).

The Influence of Hollow Fiber Dialyzer Reuse on Its Function

M. Hrubý, S. Sulková, J. Kurajský, O. Lapčík, A. Válek

Abstract

Selected parameters of dialyzer function were studied in 31 patients using reused Cuprophan hollow fiber dialyzers (HFD) and 21 patients using plate dialyzers. Reused HFD achieved sufficient urea (153.3 ± 45.8 ml/min) and creatinine (142.9 ± 41.2 ml/min) clearances. The values did not decrease under those of plate dialyzers (155.9 ± 29.3 and 141.6 ± 28.1 ml/min, respectively). Ultrafiltration ability did not change after reuse. The values of ultrafiltration coefficient (4.4 ± 1.9 ml/hour/mm Hg) remained within the required values (2 to 5 ml/hour/mm Hg). Reused HFD did not require higher heparin doses. Heparin consumption remained on the same level or even decreased after reuse. The maximal decrease of leukocyte count at 15 minutes of dialysis diminished after repeated use (51 ± 26 % at first use vs. 17 ± 15 % at more than 2nd use of HFD). Granulocytes decreased more (71 ± 21 %) than lymphocytes (36 ± 11 %). The serum concentration of β-2-microglobulin was not influenced by reuse of HFD. On the basis of our results we conclude that reused HFD are more biocompatible from the point of view of the investigated parameters and still achieve reliable efficacy.

Introduction

The growing number of hemodialysis sessions leads to increased expenditures on this mode of chronic renal replacement therapy. Among several ways how to lower the price of each dialysis, reuse, i.e. regeneration and repeated use of the same dialyser or other devices during next sessions, takes place [1, 2]. Besides the economical advantage there always emerges the problem of patients' clinical benefits under such conditions [2-6]. We have tried to prove that reuse does not negatively influence patients' well-being and the efficacy of dialyses with regenerated hollow fiber dialyzers is not deteriorated by the method used.

In our in vivo study we investigated urea and creatinine clearances, ultrafiltration coefficient, heparinization, changes in leukocyte counts and serum β-2-microglobulin (B2M) concentration, in order to assess the influence of dialyzer reuse on its function and biocompatibility.

Material and Methods

Cuprophan hollow fiber dialyzers Hemomed C1.3 (Fresenius, FRG / Hemofarm, Yugoslavia), which have the useful area of $1.3\,m^2$ and are sterilized by ethylene oxide, were used. We used dialysis monitors AK-10 equipped with ultrafiltration monitors UFM-10 (Gambro, Sweden).

Regeneration of these dialysers is done by Renatron, a machine from Renal Systems, USA. The machine regenerates one hollow fiber dialyzer within eight minutes, including performing a blood path volume test and membrane integrity test. The procedure is based on the principle of reverse ultrafiltration. The process is fully automated and performed by one of the dialysis nurses. Between dialyses the dialyzers are stored in the refrigerator at four degrees Centigrade; the sterilizing agent is 0.5 % peracetic acid.

We investigated 31 patients using HFD Hemomed. The control group consisted of 21 patients using Cuprophan plate dialyzers Chiraplat (Chirana, Czechoslovakia) with nearly the same effective membrane area ($1.4\,m^2$). Actual blood flow rate was 250-300 ml/min. Dialysate flow rate was 500 ml/min.

Calculations of urea and creatinine clearances were based on measuring their concentrations in blood and dialysate at 60 minutes of dialysis (Equation 1). Blood samples were also taken before and after dialysis to check the steady-state concentrations of the patients.

$$K_{F_u} = \frac{Q_D \cdot [u]_{Do}}{[u]_{Bi}} \qquad (1)$$

Calculation of dialyzer clearance for urea and creatinine.

u : urea or creatinine, respectively
K_{F_u} : dialyzer clearance for urea and creatinine, respectively (ml/min)
Q_D : dialysate flow rate (ml/min)
$[u]_{Do}$: concentration of urea and creatinine, respectively, in dialysate outlet (mmol/l)
$[u]_{Bi}$: concentration of urea and creatinine, respectively, in blood inlet (mmol/l)

Ultrafiltration was evaluated by the ultrafiltration coefficient (UFC) computed from ultrafiltration rate and transmembrane pressure indicated on the monitors at 60 minutes of dialysis (Equation 2).

Heparinization was described by heparin sensitivity, i.e. prolongation of pre-dialysis clotting time at the 10 minutes after administration of the initial dose of heparin, and heparin elimination constant, i.e. the relative speed of heparin elimination. These values were computed on the basis of heparin doses and values of activated clotting time, ACT, measured by Hemochron (International Technidyne, USA).

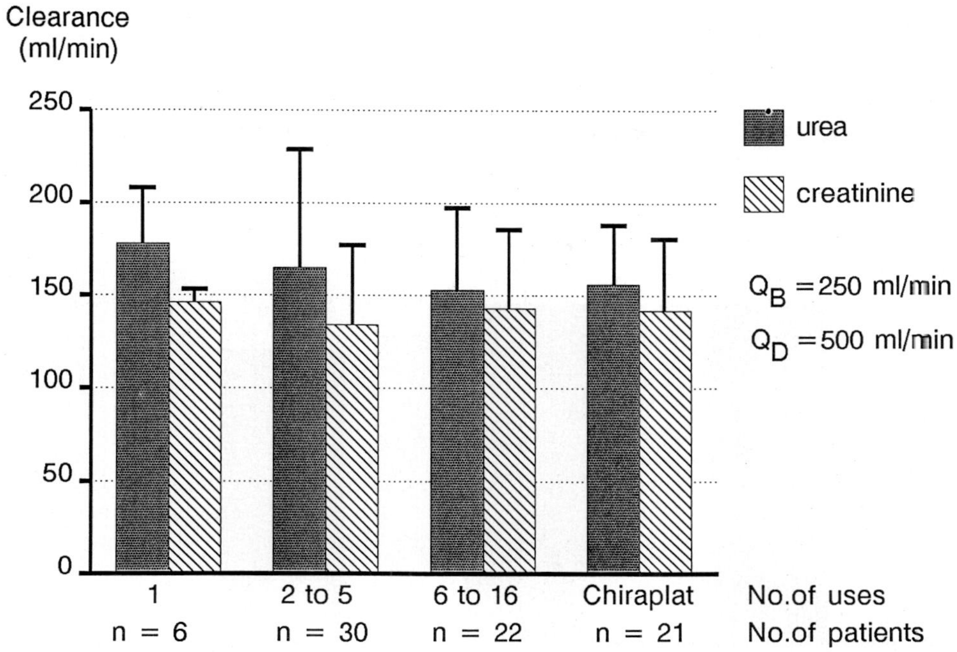

Fig. 1. Dialyzer clearances in vivo for urea and creatinine (Q_B: blood flow; Q_D: dialysate flow).

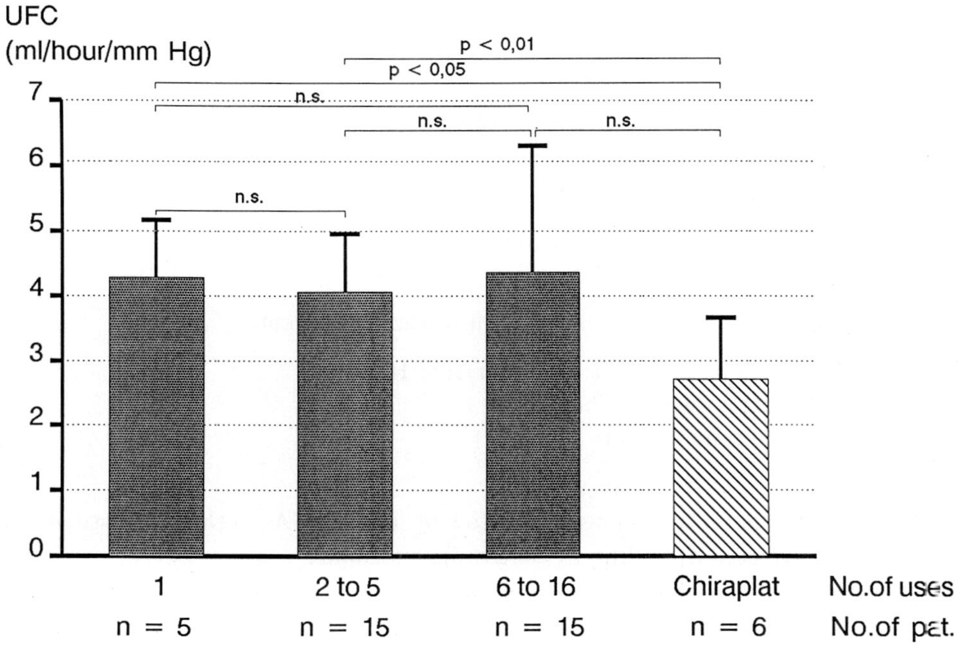

Fig. 2. Ultrafiltration coefficient (UFC).

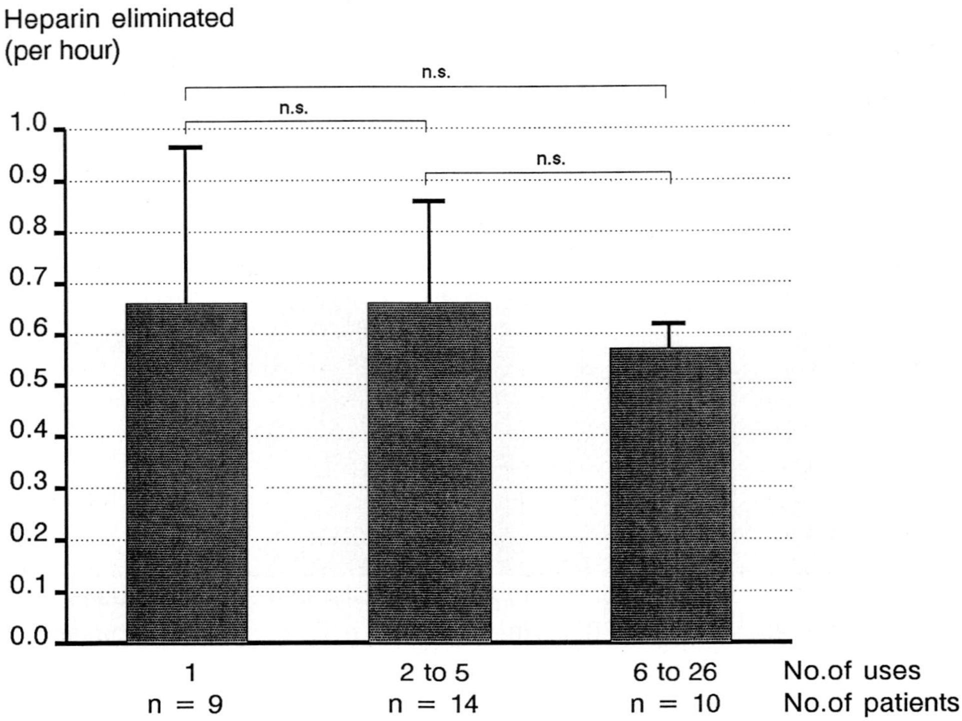

Fig. 3. Heparin elimination constant.

Both leukocytes and differential counts were counted by a single hematologist in our hematology laboratory using standard techniques.

$$\mathrm{UFC} = \frac{\mathrm{UFR}}{\mathrm{TMP}} \qquad (2)$$

Calculation of ultrafiltration coefficient.

UFC : ultrafiltration coefficient (ml/hour/mm Hg)
UFR : ultrafiltration rate (ml/hour)
TMP : transmembrane pressure (mm Hg)

Serum B2M concentration was detected by the ELISA methods. Postdialysis values were corrected according to Bergström's formula.

All patients in the study were closely watched for unwanted effects that could be manifestations of bioincompatibility of the dialysis devices [2, 6]. Bacteriological and pyrogen tests were done in the National Institute for Drug Control in Prague.

Results

Both urea and creatinine clearances achieve sufficient values even after more than five repeated uses (mean 153.3 ± 45.8 and 142.9 ± 41.2 ml/min, respectively) thus not significantly different from clearance values of the Czech plate dialyzer (155.9 ± 29.3 and 141.6 ± 28.1 ml/min, respectively) (Fig. 1).

The ultrafiltration ability, described by the UFC, fits into the required range between 2 to 5 ml of fluid removed within one hour under the transmembrane pressure of 1 mm of Hg (mean 4.4 ± 1.9 ml/hour/mm Hg after more than six uses). The changes of UFC during repeated use were not significant (Fig. 2).

The influence of dialyzer reuse on the heparinization of dialyzed patients is expressed in Figure 3 by the heparin elimination constant. Its value was 0.7 ± 0.3 per hour (mean) in the first use of the dialyzers; its change during reuse is not significant: mean 0.6 ± 0.03 after more than five uses.

The changes of leukocytes count and differential count (i.e. relative numbers of granulocytes and lymphocytes) are shown in Figures 4 and 5, respectively. With the increasing number of reuses the decrease of leukocytes at the 15 minutes of dialysis was substantially smaller, being 17 ± 15 % at more than two uses vs. 53 ± 26 % at the first use of HFD or 57 ± 20 % at plate dialyzers.

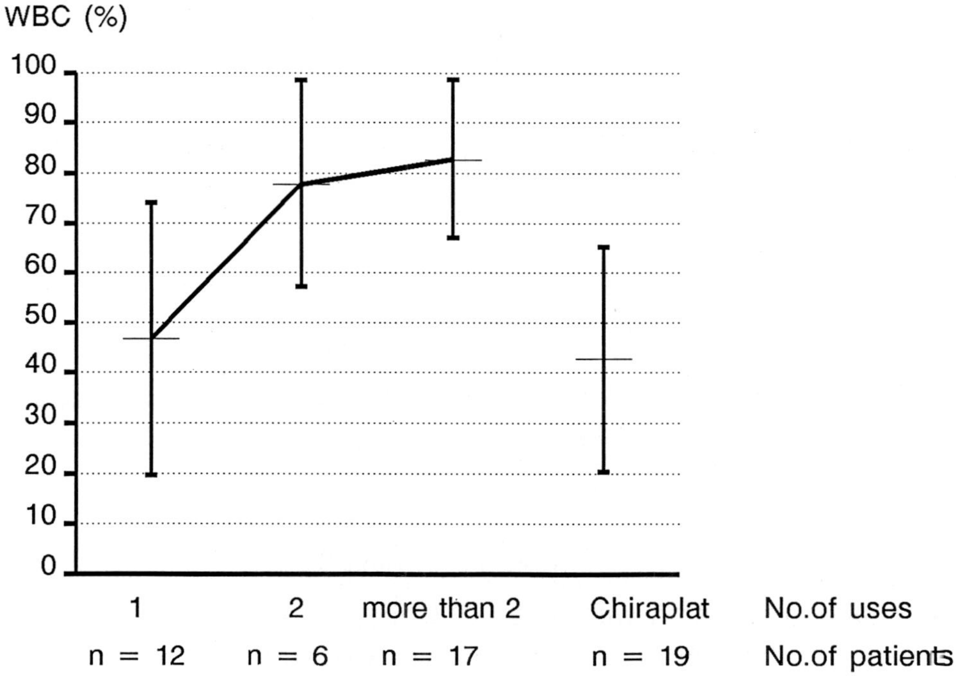

Fig. 4. White blood cells (WBC) count at the 15 minutes of hemodialysis (relative number in %).

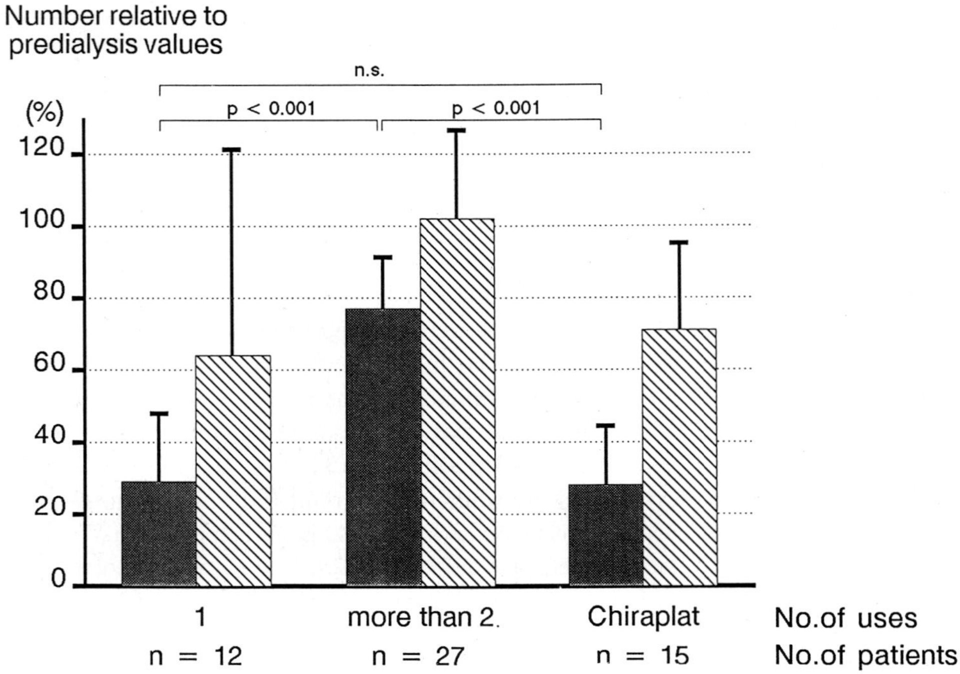

Fig. 5. Granulocytes and lymphocytes at the 15 minutes of hemodialysis.

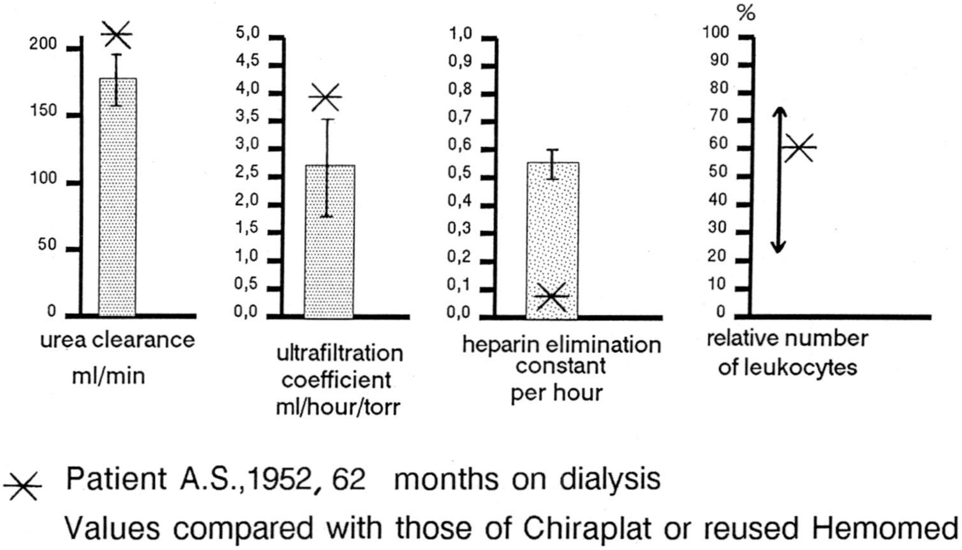

Fig. 6. The efficacy of hollow fiber dialyzer during 36th use.

However, serum β-2-microglobulin concentration was not influenced by regeneration and reuse of dialyzers. Both with the first use and reused HFD its value increased during dialysis: from 36.5 ± 16.0 μg/l to 43.6 ± 17.3 μg/l at first use and from 37.0 ± 17.4 μg/l to 44.3 ± 19.3 μg/l after reuse of HFD. These differences are not significant (Table 1).

Table 1. Serum β-2-microglobulin (B2M) concentration after reuse.

No. of use	No. of patients	Serum B2M concentration (μg/l)	
		predialysis	postdialysis
1	20	29.3 ± 13.99	34.5 ± 11.22
≥ 2	10	31.3 ± 14.6	34.8 ± 15.8

There was a patient who used one HFD for 36 consequent dialyses. The values of all measured parameters proved sufficient efficacy of the dialyzer even after its 36th use. When compared with plate dialysers or reused Hemomeds, all the values reached the required levels or were even better (Fig. 6). After the 36th use the dialyzer was discarded only for ethical reasons.

Discussion

We have confirmed that reuse of HFD does not lead to significant decrease of urea and/or creatinine clearances in vivo [2, 4, 7]. The mean values of clearances of HFD (153.3 ± 45.8 ml/min for urea and 142.9 ± 41.2 ml/min for creatinine) after more than five uses did not differ significantly from the mean values of plate dialyzers (155.9 ± 29.3 ml/min and 141.6 ± 28.1 ml/min, respectively).

The ultrafiltration ability may be described by the so called UFC, which represents the amount of fluid removed per one hour under one unit of transmembrane pressure (TMP) [8]. During reuse, theoretically, it could increase due to microdisruptions of the membrane, or decrease as a consequence of blood clotting in membrane pores [2]. UFC should reach values between 2-5 ml/hour/mm Hg [9]. The value of UFC of reused HFD meets this requirement, with the mean value of 4.4 ± 1.9 ml/hour/mm Hg after numerous reuses. Opposite to clearances, the value of UFC did not decrease; its changes are not significant.

What about heparinization? Is there any need to increase the doses of the heparin during dialyses with reused dialyzers? Based on our investigation of the heparin elimination constant, there is no need to increase the dosage of heparin as anticoagulant agent for dialyses with reused dialysers. The heparin elimination constant, i.e. the relative speed of heparin consumption during dialysis [8], remained on the same level or even decreased (mean 0.7 ± 0.3 at first use and 0.6 ± 0.03 after more than five uses). This trend was also seen while determining the heparin elimination constant during consequent dialyses at several patients.

We followed the changes of leukocytes counts during dialysis as an expression of membrane biocompatibility. Maximal decrease of the values appeared at the 15 minutes of dialysis, as expected [10, 11]. During 1st use of HFD the decrease was comparable with our findings for plate dialyzers with the same membrane material (means $53 \pm 26\,\%$ and $57 \pm 20\,\%$, respectively). After reuse, the decrease was substantially smaller (mean $17 \pm 15\,\%$ after more than two uses). Granulocytes are responsible for this phenomenon more than other leukocytes: the decrease was $72 \pm 16\,\%$ of their predialysis level at plate dialyzers and $71 \pm 21\,\%$ at first use of HFD. After more than two uses of HFD the decrease of granulocytes was significantly different ($23 \pm 28\,\%$ mean). On the contrary, lymphocytes were lowered much less ($36 \pm 11\,\%$) or even increased from their predialysis level [11].

Serum β-2-microglobulin concentration during Cuprophan dialysis increases. It was suggested that this increase may be due to bioincompatibility of this membrane [12-14]. In our study, during hemodialysis with first used dialyzers serum B2M concentration increased regularly. However, a similar increase was observed also during dialysis with reused HFD. We suggest that regeneration of dialyzers does not influence serum B2M and that its concentration changes are not a marker of biocompatibility [15-17].

Conclusions

On the basis of our results it may be concluded:

Regeneration and reuse of hollow fiber dialyzers is an economically advantageous mode of chronic dialysis treatment.

Reused HFD achieve sufficient urea and creatinine clearances.

The ultrafiltration coefficient does not change during reuse.

Reuse of HFD does not require a change in heparin doses.

β-2-microglobulin concentration changes during reuse did not differ from those observed with plate dialyzers or new hollow fiber dialyzers.

The maximal drop of leukocyte count is much less pronounced in reused HFD than in new ones. Granulocytes are more responsible for this decrease than lymphocytes. From the point of view of the investigated parameters reused HFD are more biocompatible than new ones.

Acknowledgements

Special thanks to Professor Albert Válek, M.D., Ph.D., for the kindest support in everything concerning this topics.

References

[1] FOXEN, L. G.: Is reuse cost effective? A case study. *Dial Transplant* 13(5): 290-293 (1984).

[2] DEANE, N., J. A. BEMIS: Multiple use of hemodialyzers, pp. 286-304. In: DRUKKER, W., F. M. PARSONS, J. F. MAHER (eds.): Replacement of renal function by dialysis. Martinus Nijhoff Publ.: Boston 1983.

[3] CHAROENPANICH, R., V. E. POLLAK, K. S. KANT, M. D. ROBSON, M. CATHEY: Effect of first and subsequent use of hemodialyzers on patient well-being: the rise and fall of a syndrome associated with new dialyzer use. *Art. Organs* 11(2): 123-127 (1987).

[4] CHURCHILL, D. N., D. W. TAYLOR, A. G. SHIMIZU, M. L. BEECROFT, J. SINGER, D. LUDWIN, C. C. BARNES, N. WRIGHT, D. L. SACKETT, E. K. M. SMITH: Dialyzer reuse – a multiple crossover study with random allocation to order of treatment. *Nephron* 50: 325-331 (1988).

[5] KLINKMANN, H.: Invited summary and conclusions. *Dial. Transplant.* 16(1): 34 (1987).

[6] VANHOLDER, R., S. RINGOIR: Influence of reuse and reuse sterilants on the first-use syndrome. *Art. Organs* 11(2): 137-139 (1987).

[7] VILLARROEL, F.: First-use syndrome in patients treated with hollow-fiber dialyzers. *Blood Purific.* 5: 112-114 (1987).

[8] SARGENT, J. A., F. A. GOTCH: Principles and biophysics of dialysis, pp. 53-96. In: DRUKKER, W., F. M. PARSONS, J. F. MAHER (eds.): Replacement of renal function by dialysis. Martinus Nijhoff Publ.: Boston 1983.

[9] HOENICH, N. A., D. N. S. KERR: Dialyzers, pp. 104-141. In: DRUKKER, W., F. M. PARSONS, J. F. MAHER (eds.): Replacement of renal function by dialysis. Martinus Nijhoff Publ.: Boston 1983.

[10] HÖRL, W. H., W. RIEGEL, H. B. STEINHAUER, C. WANNER, F. THAISS, F. BOZKURT, M. HAAG, P. SCHOLLMEYER: Granulocyte activation during hemodialysis. *Clin. Nephr.* 26 (Suppl.1): 30-34 (1986).

[11] JØRSTAD, S.: Biocompatibility of different hemodialysis and plasmapheresis membranes. *Blood Purific.* 5: 123-137 (1987).

[12] DEUBER, H. J., H. G. MÜHLBAUER , W. SCHULZ, R. FRANK: β-2-microglobulin as indicator of biocompatibility of different dialysator membrane material. In: Abstracts from 5th Annual Meeting of the International Society of Blood Purification. *Blood Purific.* 5: 278 (1987).

[13] DRÜECKE, T., J. ZINGRAFF, P. UREÑA, G. JEHENNE, N. K. MAN: Plasma β-2-microglobulin (B2-M) changes induced by different dialysis membranes. In: Abstracts from 5th Annual Meeting of the International Society of Blood Purification. *Blood Purific.* 5:279 (1987).

[14] WIDERØE, T. E., T. BALSTAD, S. JØRSTAD, L. C. SMEBY, K. DAHL: Comparison between dialyzer membrane biocompatibility in vitro and in vivo. In: Abstracts from 5th Annual Meeting of the International Society of Blood Purification. *Blood Purific.* 5: 317 (1987).

[15] COLTON, C. K.: Technical foundations of renal prosthesis, pp. 187-218. In: GURLAND, H. J. (ed.): Uremia therapy. Perspectives for the next quarter century. Springer: Berlin 1987.

[16] GRANOLLERAS, C., S. DESCHODT, S. SHALDON, J. FLÖGE, K. M. KOCH, P. J. KNUDSEN, C. K. COLTON: The rise of plasma β-2-microglobulin (B2-m) during cuprophan hemodialysis is real but is not due to cuprophan per se. In: Abstracts from 5th Annual Meeting of the International Society of Blood Purification. *Blood Purific.* 5: 285 (1987).

[17] BERGSTRÖM, J., B. WEHLE: Plasma β-2-microglobulin (B2M) concentration before and after hemodialysis (HD) with eight different dialyzers. In: Abstracts from 5th Annual Meeting of the International Society of Blood Purification. *Blood Purific.* 5: 316 (1987).

Index